FIT
AT
50

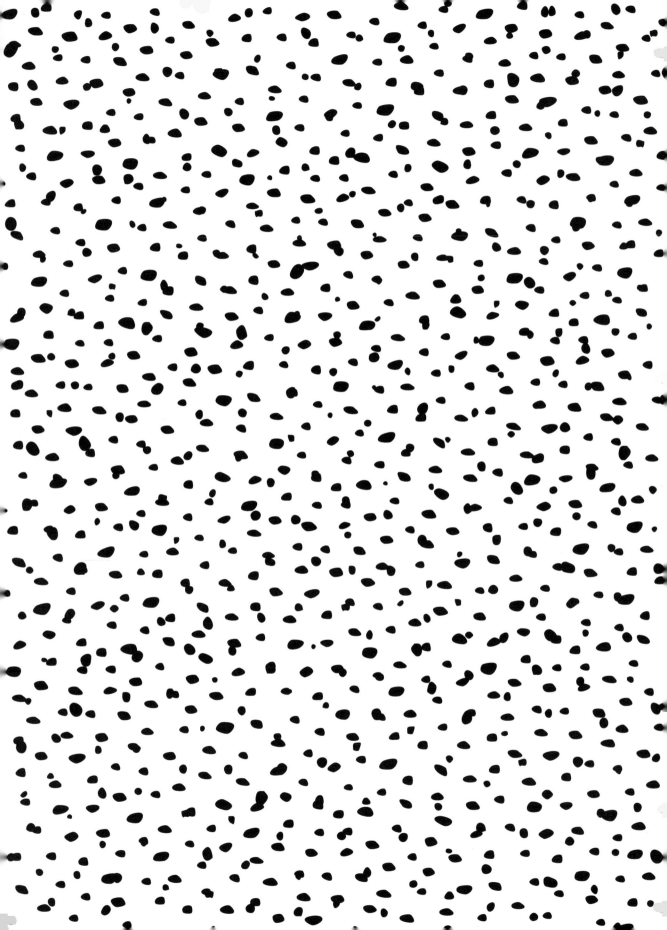

CAROLINE IDIENS

FIT AT 50

YOUR GUIDE TO A STRONGER, FITTER
& HAPPIER (MID)LIFE IN JUST 6 WEEKS

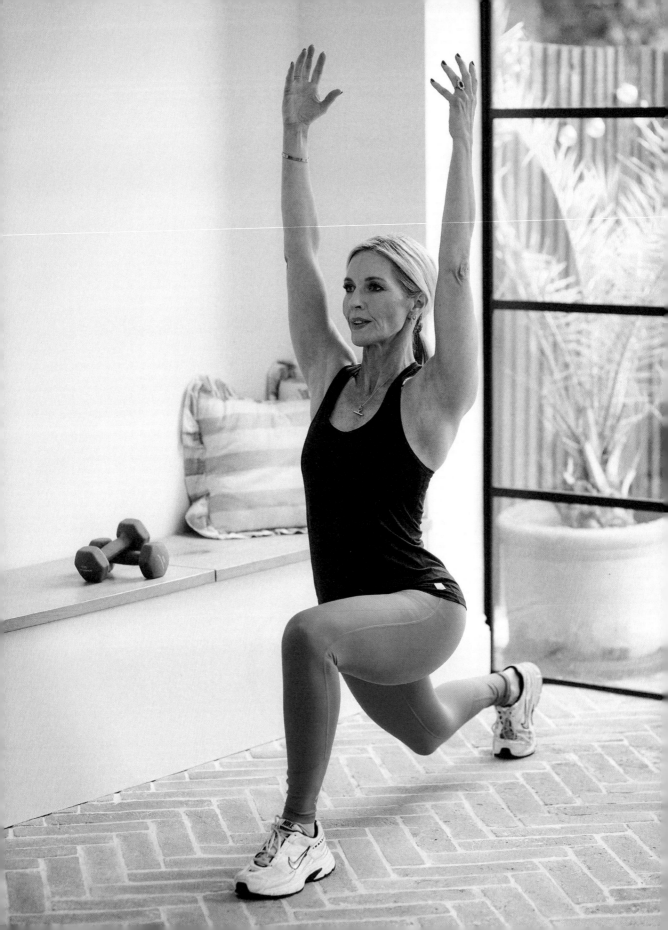

CONTENTS

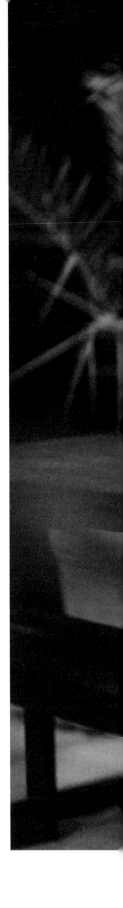

WELCOME.

I'm Caroline, a mother of two and the founder of Caroline's Circuits, an online fitness platform dedicated to strength workouts. Many of you may know me from my online classes or social media, but I'm so excited to share with you my whole 360-degree approach behind what you see on the screen. In this book I will break down everything I have learned as a trainer—all the valuable knowledge and techniques I have accumulated over 25 years and that have changed my life and those of my clients. As your coach, I want to motivate, help, and encourage you to discover the joy of exercising and being strong in midlife. To make small lifestyle changes that will truly transform your health and well-being. This is much more than yet another exercise manual or a promise of a quick fix. This is about *prioritizing you*! While it's a book about midlife, it is also a book for women of *all* ages—for our daughters, our granddaughters, our friends, and our colleagues. It's about strong women and the pillars or foundations that make us so.

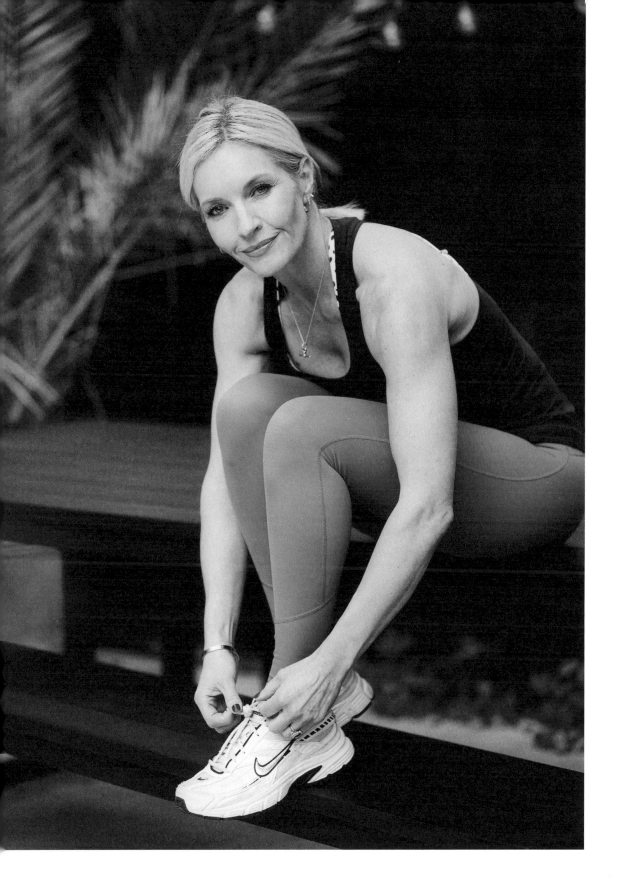

"I GENUINELY LOOK FORWARD TO DOING CAROLINE'S WORKOUTS AS I KNOW THAT I WILL FEEL 100% BETTER AFTERWARD."

I am genuinely passionate about what you are about to read. This is a six-week plan with goals that are achievable. The exercise program, simple meals, advice, and practical tips will improve your daily life, mood, and overall fitness and, in the long term, ensure a stronger future.

I have worked as a personal trainer throughout my career. Over the past 20 years, I have seen the fitness landscape change so much. Throughout my twenties and thirties, it was all about the calorie burn, the aesthetics, the crazy diet, meals on the run, and exercise programs that were simply not viable in the long-term. I spent little time on strength workouts—the emphasis was always on cardio. However, as we grow older, with the shift in hormones and decline in muscle and bone health, this way of exercising just isn't sustainable. Instead, the emphasis should be on building a stronger body, enjoying a more nutritious diet, a better night's sleep, and prioritizing wellness as a whole. Not only for physical strength, but mental strength too.

My vision for this book, as well as for my online platform, is to reframe and refocus the way that we view our lifestyle habits, especially during this midlife period. So many women feel lost at this stage of their lives; unseen, unheard, and quite often lacking in confidence. I want to show women how to discover a new confidence in their bodies and a newfound strength at a time in their lives when self-esteem might be lacking. We can draw on years of experience and be "fit at 50," showing the world that this is actually a fabulous time in our lives. This book will show you how to do this—by keeping everything simple, consistent, and focusing on our mindset as much as our movement.

I've collaborated with a fantastic dietitian, Laura Clark, to bring you recipes that are realistic and not restrictive, alongside workouts that are challenging yet easily done in the comfort of your own home.

I believe that it is all about making sustainable choices for long-term results. I am here to give you practical and achievable ways in which you can change your lifestyle by tweaking your everyday choices and building long-term habits. I'm doing this *with you*. I am a woman in midlife with a busy, hectic lifestyle too. We can do this together; to be fit at 40, at 50, as well as at 60, 70, and beyond! Midlife is about prioritizing *you*; this is our time to shine.

HOW TO USE THIS BOOK

I want this book to be viewed as a toolkit for success, with a focus on the following:

1   BACK TO BASICS
What are your goals? How are you feeling and what do you want to take away from this book? Is there balance in your life? Write it down!

2   WHAT'S REALLY IMPORTANT?
The key pillars to leading a healthy lifestyle: exercise, nutrition, sleep, mindset.

3   THE SIX-WEEK EXERCISE PLAN
All you need to get started. A plan with step-by-step instructions for each exercise and a six-week program for building strength. With modifications, advice on weights, and information for preventing injuries, I have it all covered! Plus, I look at ways to warm up and cool down so that you can exercise safely.

4   NOURISHING NUTRITION
From trusted nutritional information from a registered dietitian to suggestions of daily meal plans and delicious recipes, learn how to fuel your body for optimum results.

5   WHERE DO YOU GO FROM HERE?
My top tips going forward. What's next? See how far you've come, how to sustain it, and continue progressing!

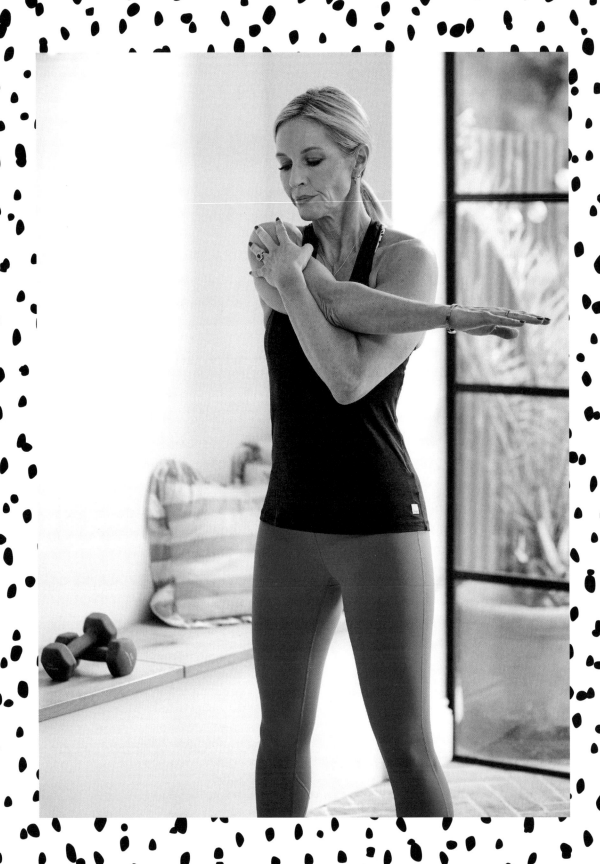

BACK TO
BASICS

Let's start at the beginning. My six-week strength program, alongside delicious recipes, will show you ways to make long-term improvements to your health.

This is not a "new you" book; this is an exercise and nutrition guide that we will work through together—finding ways to make healthy lifestyle changes with small daily steps. You may have seen exercise and meal plans before and thought, "There's no way I can do that!" My program is different. It's not about quick fixes, bikini bodies, and calorie-counting meals. Instead, I want us to form healthy habits together, which will make a fundamental difference as we age. My six-week exercise plan is built on resistance-based circuits using minimal equipment, with step-by-step guides for each movement so that you can easily follow them at home. Starting with 20–25-minute sessions, these are workouts that fit into everyday life and—most importantly—*your* life. These exercises are the ones that I live by and that have worked not only for me but also for my clients for the past 20 years.

The workouts are then accompanied by recipes to nourish and fuel your body. From delicious snacks and smoothies, to main meals that work for the whole family. I have clients now in their forties, fifties, and sixties who are healthier, fitter, and happier than they were in their twenties and thirties. It's never too late to make changes to improve your health.

It's also important to consider what's happening in midlife. Menopause comes with a myriad of symptoms and changes that might not all be welcome. These range from surreptitious weight gain, joint aches and pains, to the dreaded hot flashes, general lethargy, anxiety, and mood swings. However, one thing that has been proven time and time again is how exercise and a healthy diet can help at this stage of life and make a huge difference in how we feel both physically and mentally.

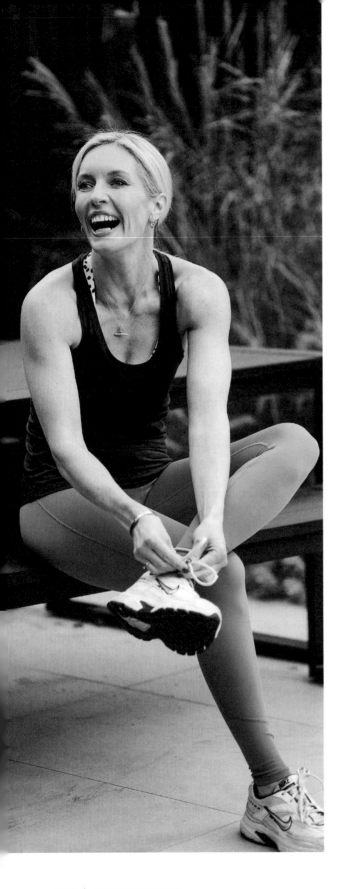

WHERE DO I START?

Motivation? Willpower? Is this enough to make the changes that you need? Just as brushing your teeth or washing your hands are part of your daily routine, I want to show you how small, sustainable lifestyle changes can make a huge difference in how you feel long-term.

We lead hectic, modern lifestyles where we are used to quick fixes. Before starting the plan, it is important to take a step back and look at our busy lives. I call it a 360-degree approach, looking at your life from every angle.

WHAT DO WELL-BEING AND BALANCE MEAN TO YOU DURING MIDLIFE?

Take five minutes to pause and think about the questions on the following page. Try to reflect on your current lifestyle and routine. There are no right or wrong answers; everyone is different. Finding balance is key, so take a moment at the start of this book to think about what it means to you and for *your* life.

> "I'M A BEGINNER AND I'M AMAZED AT HOW MUCH FITTER I'VE BECOME IN JUST THREE MONTHS."

SOME QUESTIONS TO ASK YOURSELF BEFORE YOU BEGIN

EXERCISE

Do you exercise?

How important is exercise in your daily life?

Is it something you enjoy or something you dread?

NUTRITION

What does your diet look like?

What do you eat on a daily basis?

How regular are your mealtimes?

Do you eat on the go?

Do you eat with family?

Do you like to cook from scratch?

How much water do you drink?

SLEEP

How much sleep do you get on an average night?

What quality of sleep do you get?

Do you eat late at night?

Is your screen time affecting your sleep?

MINDSET

Do you check in with yourself on a regular basis?

Are you happy?

Do you enjoy time outside?

What makes you smile?

Do you keep a journal?

YOUR EXPERIENCE OF MIDLIFE

Are you suffering with menopausal symptoms?

Do you have joint pain?

Do you have headaches, stress, or anxiety?

Do you think about your gut health?

Do you want to feel stronger?

THE
FOUR PILLARS

Balance can be achieved by addressing the four fundamental pillars that are crucial for longevity.

EXERCISE

Exercise is hugely beneficial, not only for our physical health, but for our mental health, too. Exercise strengthens our muscles, bones, brains, and hearts and reduces our risk of disease. At the same time, it boosts our confidence, mood, and focus.

NUTRITION

A balanced diet is fundamental to a healthy and long life providing all the nutrients we need to support our bodies on a daily basis. It fuels us, supports our immunity, improves mental clarity, and reduces the risk of chronic disease.

SLEEP

Sleep is essential for our physical and mental well-being. Not only does it allow the body to repair, recover, and rejuvenate, but it is also vital for our focus, mood, and immunity.

MINDSET

A positive mindset can have a beneficial impact on our physical as well as our mental well-being. It encourages us to make healthier lifestyle choices, cope with challenges and stress more effectively, and keeps us motivated and fulfilled as we age.

SETTING GOALS

Finding balance requires giving yourself sustainable targets to work toward.

The exercise program in this book enables you to do as little or as much as your life allows. Here are a few top tips for how to set goals:

1 **Start small** Consistency is your best friend. Small changes will gently adjust habits and allow for long-term results. This applies as much to the food you eat as to your fitness goals. Remember—changes take time.

2 **Think long-term** How much time do you have to achieve your ultimate goal? Is it to feel happier and fitter? Or more confident in midlife?

3 **Find something you enjoy!** It's then much more likely that you will stick with it. My exercise plan gives you a framework and the flexibility to exercise when you can fit it into your everyday routine. Maybe you can do a 15-minute stretch before heading out for the day. If you can try and connect a new habit to an existing habit that is an excellent start—for example, while you are running a bath you could be doing your tricep dips!

4 **Find a space that is yours and own that time and the environment** There may be a particular time slot that works for you; energize your morning with a short 10-minute cardio blast or bookmark your day with a post-work stretch.

5 **These simple tips may also help:**
   - Seize the day and start early
   - Get outside for a walk before breakfast
   - Lay out your exercise clothes the night before
   - Set your alarm 20 minutes earlier
   - Arrange to meet a friend for a walk or schedule a workout class together
   - Write your workouts down and keep track of your progress
   - Don't try to do everything at once. Build up gradually and you are more likely to keep going

EXERCISE
AND MIDLIFE

Not everyone will go through perimenopause or menopause in the same way, but we need to help ourselves as best we can during this time. Incorporating regular exercise into your daily routine can lead to significant improvements in your overall health and well-being.

WHY EXERCISE NOW?

As a woman in my fifties, I find that the benefits of exercising regularly are countless—I cannot imagine my life without movement. So why is exercise—and particularly strength training—so important at this time?

Maintaining and building muscle mass As women age, they experience a natural decline in muscle mass and strength, a condition known as sarcopenia. It typically begins around the age of 30 and can accelerate after the age of 60. Strength training helps to counteract this decline by stimulating muscle growth and maintenance, which is essential for overall physical health and functionality. Keeping our muscles strong will help to keep us injury-free, maintaining the ability to perform everyday activities with ease.

Improving bone density From the age of 35, our bone density decreases, and by midlife, as estrogen levels decline, women develop a greater risk of osteoporosis. In the first five years post-menopause, women can lose up to 10% of their bone mass. Osteoporosis is characterized by weakened bones and it increases the probability of fractures. Strength training promotes new bone-cell growth and helps to retain bone density, reducing the risk of fractures. Try low-impact exercises in your routine where there will be less stress on the joints. These include cycling, swimming, and walking alongside strength training.

Improving bone and joint movement As we approach midlife, and especially from the age of 40, we need to focus more attention on our joints as well as our bones. As we age, joint movement becomes stiffer and less flexible due to the decrease of lubricating fluid inside the joints and the cartilage becoming thinner (osteoarthritis). Ligaments also tend to shorten and lose some flexibility, making joints feel stiff. Strength training targets individual muscle groups and strengthens the muscles around the joints, helping to take the pressure off them. It can also improve the flow of nutrients to the cartilage. Functional training will help joints move freely, improve mobility, and therefore help in daily activities, preventing injuries as we age—find out more on pages 36–37.

Retaining our balance and mobility Posture, mobility, and coordination can decline as we get older, and we can therefore face an increased risk of falls and injury. Strengthening our core muscles as well as other muscle groups through resistance training will not only improve our posture but will stabilize the body, reducing the strain on our back. Strong core muscles help us with our balance and enable us to perform day-to-day tasks trouble-free.

Managing weight and reducing body fat

Hormonal changes during midlife can cause our metabolism to slow, and reduced estrogen levels alter fat storage patterns, which shift fat accumulation from the hips and thighs to the belly. Strength training boosts muscle mass, which in turn increases your basic metabolic rate (BMR). A higher BMR means that the body burns more calories at rest, aiding weight management and fat loss.

Achieving better cardiovascular health

Preventing cardiovascular diseases, keeping cholesterol levels in check, and maintaining good circulation are all things we have to keep in mind during midlife and beyond. Cardio exercises such as running have traditionally been emphasized as great for maintaining cardiovascular health, but strength training also plays a crucial role in reducing blood pressure and improving cholesterol levels. Combining strength training with regular aerobic exercise will ensure that your heart stays healthy.

Enhancing our mental well-being Due to a combination of hormonal, physical, and emotional changes, our stress levels often increase during perimenopause and menopause. Exercise releases endorphins, the chemicals in the brain that act as natural painkillers and mood elevators. Strength training is particularly effective at reducing cortisol levels. Cortisol is a hormone produced by the adrenal glands in response to stress. Regular strength training can help the body become more efficient at reducing cortisol levels, combatting stress, and promoting better mental health.

Supporting immunity As the body ages, the immune system naturally begins to decline, making it increasingly important to adopt habits that support our immune function. By keeping us active and healthy, strength training helps bolster the immune system and ensures it is better equipped to ward off illnesses.

Improving sleep quality Midlife is often associated with interrupted sleep and insomnia. Hormonal fluctuations during perimenopause and menopause can lead to night sweats, hot flashes, and general discomfort, which can disrupt our sleep. Strength training can help regulate hormones, reduce stress, and manage weight—all factors that can affect our sleep. Exercise will also improve sleep quality, which in turn supports immunity, enhances our mood, and increases our energy levels for the following day.

FUTURE-PROOF YOUR BODY

The strength training workouts in my book target individual muscle groups as well as compound movements, which will help to future-proof your bones and joints. Staying active is actually one of the best things you can do for your long-term health:

- **Start with body-weight exercises instead of heavy weights.** Exercises using body weight only include squats (see page 54) and lunges (see page 65).
- **Flexibility exercises are key.** Ensure you always warm up for 5–10 minutes before exercising with dynamic stretches rather than static exercises to loosen up the joints, improve circulation, and prepare the body for exercise. I have included examples of these in the program.
- **Correct posture, alignment, and good balance will help protect your joints and prevent falls and instability.** I have included core strengthening exercises throughout the program to help you with this.
- **Skeletal muscle plays a vital role in everything we do**—it is essential that we maintain it for our future health.
- **Don't forget the glutes!** Strengthening the glutes may help prevent lower back pain, correct your alignment, improve your posture and balance, and boost your performance overall.

"I TURNED 50 LAST WEEK, I HAVE MUSCLES I DIDN'T KNOW EXISTED, AND I FEEL STRONGER, FITTER AND LEANER THAN EVER."

DO SHORT WORKOUTS WORK?

The answer is…YES! The workouts in this book are all 30 minutes or less.

Sometimes it can feel daunting to begin a new exercise routine and, so, if you are struggling for motivation it's helpful to remember that short workouts really are effective for many reasons. All movement counts and small bursts really add up.

FIND YOUR FOCUS

First, you're much more likely to stay focused in a shorter time period. It's all about quality over quantity. If you can do 10–15 minutes of good-quality exercise, you will have better concentration, as well as being able to fit it into your daily life.

Short workouts are also a great way to build activity into your day, which will then, in turn, kick-start a new habit. What starts out as a short session can slowly become a regular habit and long-term lifestyle change.

KEEP MOTIVATED

Shorter workouts are brilliant for motivation and getting started. Remember that if you're only spending 10/15/20 minutes on exercise, make sure it's something that gets the heart rate up and raises your metabolism. Body-weight strength classes are excellent for this. You don't need any equipment and you can put together a basic circuit, which is easy to do at home.

For example, you could spend 5 minutes on mobility stretches at your desk, improving flexibility. Alternatively, you could focus on one muscle group at a time. Ten minutes in the morning on the upper body and ten minutes in the afternoon on legs. Or even a cardio burst with five HIIT exercises rotated.

These micro-workouts have so many health benefits, such as improving your blood sugar levels and heart health. Make sure they are something you enjoy, since you are then much more likely to stick with them. Gardening, carrying groceries, climbing stairs, and household chores and activities are all steps that count. Try dips while watching a favorite show or walking lunges around the yard. These little adaptations to your daily routine can change habits forever!

Keep it brief, but at the same time, keep it regular and consistent. While your long-term goal could be 30 minutes of exercise (as in this book), a shorter time frame is a great starting point.

Set yourself a challenge and see what you can achieve!

NUTRITION IN MIDLIFE

Eating well in midlife is about enjoying our meals and ensuring we fuel our bodies correctly, especially when our needs are changing.

One of the fundamental pillars of my plan is nutrition. I've worked with Laura Clark, a registered dietitian who specializes in providing support during midlife and menopause, to help us to eat well in our fifties.

It's crucial to understand the impact of what we eat on our overall health and fitness. The phrase "you can't outrun a bad diet" has resonated with me throughout my training career. While exercise is essential for maintaining good physical and mental health and can aid in weight management, it cannot compensate for a poor diet. This is especially important at a time when your body composition and nutritional needs are changing, such as during menopause.

This is not a time for restriction or calorie counting. The right balance of foods is essential to fuel our bodies in midlife, which we've taken care to integrate throughout the recipe section on pages 142–233. Let's dig into the fundamentals.

THE FUNDAMENTALS

1 **CARBOHYDRATES** help to regulate our blood glucose throughout the day. Whole-grain carbs tend to release energy more slowly and are also great for protecting against the increased post-menopause risk of cardiovascular disease. Fibrous carbs also provide nutrition for our gut bacteria, helping them to thrive and support us, and are often a source of protein too.

2 **POWERFUL PROTEIN** is essential for repairing muscles and bones. (See page 21 for more detailed information about protein.)

3 **HEALTHY FATS** are crucial for heart and brain health, as well as for supporting hormone production. You'll see lots of sources of omega-3 fats in my recipes, which also play a role in reducing inflammation. Including a balance of fats in your diet will help with satiety and taste satisfaction, which can reduce snack cravings.

4 **FIBROUS FOODS** help to maintain a healthy gut microbiome, which can play a crucial role in managing menopause-related symptoms, including weight gain and anxiety. As we age and go through the menopausal transition, the diversity in our gut microbiome reduces. Considering how we can support our gut through a range of different fibers is key to improving overall well-being.

5 **VITAMINS AND MINERALS** Micronutrients such as iron, calcium, and magnesium are essential for optimal body composition, protection against disease, and cellular function as we age. I'm particularly interested in bone health, and the role exercise plays to strengthen and guard against age-related bone loss, so many of my recipes contain "bone-supporting" foods. Vitamin D is needed to absorb calcium and magnesium into our bones and is a supplement you'll need in addition to your diet.

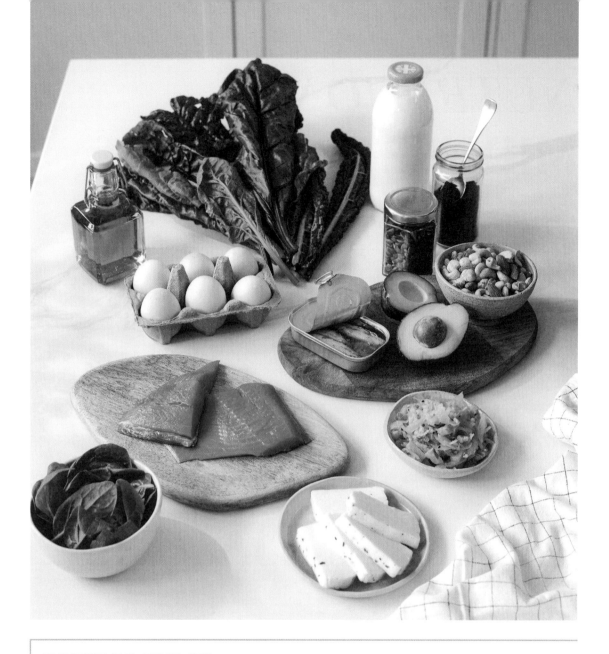

WHERE TO FIND IT?

1 **CARBOHYDRATES:** Cereals, bread, pasta, rice, noodles (whole-grain varieties where possible), quinoa, potatoes

2 **POWERFUL PROTEIN:**
- **Animal-based proteins:** Eggs, red and white meat, fish, milk, Greek yogurt
- **Plant-based proteins:** Pulses, lentils, nuts, seeds, soy e.g. tofu, tempeh

3 **HEALTHY FATS:** Avocados, olive oil, nuts, seeds, oily fish

4 **FIBROUS FOODS:** Fruit, vegetables, pulses, whole-grains

5 **VITAMINS AND MINERALS:**
- **Magnesium:** Avocado, spinach, nuts, seeds
- **Iron:** Beef, shellfish, dark leafy greens
- **Calcium:** Canned fish, dairy, tofu, broccoli
- **Vitamin D:** Oily fish, eggs
- **Omega-3:** Oily fish, flaxseed, walnuts

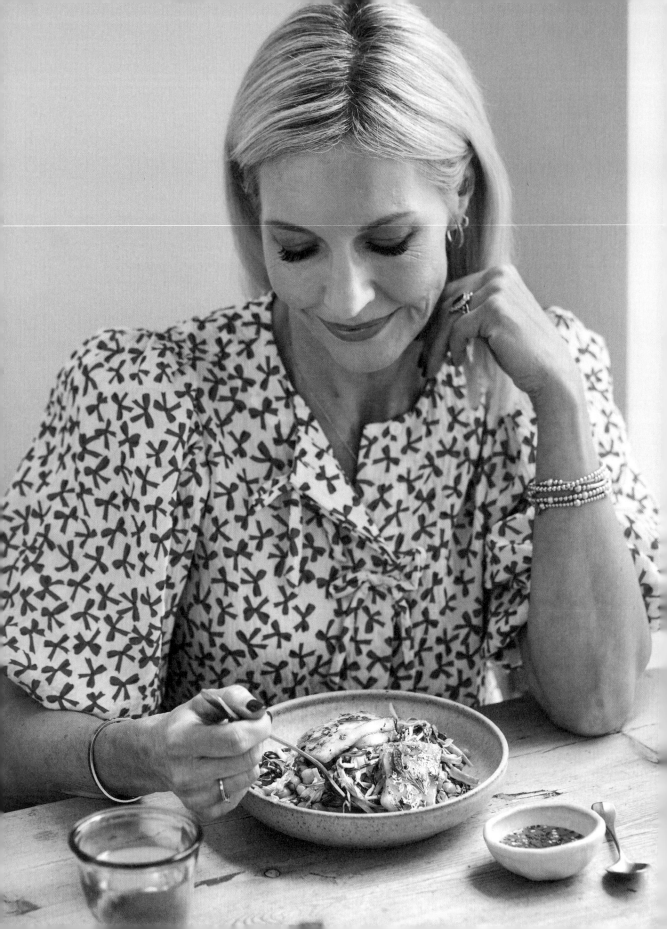

THE IMPORTANCE OF PROTEIN

The World Health Organization (WHO) recommends that healthy adults consume 0.83g of protein per kilogram of body weight per day to meet our basic requirements. However, research suggests that there are benefits to consuming 1–1.2g/kg body weight as we get older, to help prevent age-related bone loss and loss of lean muscle mass, which is accelerated as we lose estrogen in menopause.

How much protein do I need? I don't calculate my protein intake on a daily basis, because I know if I aim for a good source of protein in my meals and snacks (especially if my snacks are shortly before or after I train) that I'll be getting enough. The combination of protein with resistance training increases the benefits to our muscles and bones. Within the meal plans on page 146, I suggest a workable protein range of around 70–95g/day, because it's important to take into consideration that we'll all have slightly different requirements, but also to note how easy it can be to meet them.

When should I eat protein? Our body cannot store protein, so regulating our intake across the day is the best way to support our muscles to use it efficiently. As a guide, aim for approximately 20g of protein per meal and include a source of protein in your snacks.

Balancing our protein needs As you will see, the recipes in this book tell you how much protein and carbohydrate they contain. I wanted to show how simple it can be to combine these two macro-nutrients together to create delicious meals that also enable our bodies to function well.

There are often misunderstandings about how much protein we really need, and fears around carbohydrates. But it's important to remember that adequate fueling enables the protein we eat to be used for its primary roles, which are to build and repair body tissues such as bones and muscles, drive metabolic reactions through the production of enzymes and hormones, and ensure a strong immune system.

Eating too much protein is unnecessary and may make it harder to take on board enough fiber or fuel, and it's including these nutrients in harmony that gives us the biggest benefits for health and fitness in midlife. In practical terms, we really don't need to be consuming more than 100g of protein a day.

Types of protein The building blocks of protein are called amino acids and there are 20 that we need, nine of which are "essential" because they cannot be made in our bodies and must be provided by our diet. Animal-based proteins contain all the essential amino acids, while plant-based proteins contain only some. Combining different plant-based proteins ensures we still get our full quota, and these do have some additional benefits for midlife.

Food is often said to be able to balance our hormones, but this isn't strictly true. Individual foods are not able to influence hormone levels; rather, it's the role of the body, with its intricate systems, that balances them for us. The way we can ensure this balance takes place is to create lifestyle habits that support our bodies at every stage. These are the interwoven pillars you will see highlighted in this book.

WHAT ARE THE HEALTH BENEFITS OF A BALANCED DIET?

I try to place nourishing food at the heart of my day as much as I can. If we allow our body permission to taste and savor food, our internal weight regulation systems work well for us. In my experience, calories don't paint the full picture and I don't believe in the concept of earning or burning our calories through exercise. Instead, I want to inspire you to foster a healthy, happy relationship with both eating and training that works in synergy together to make you stronger and healthier. So how does a balanced diet benefit us?

Provides essential nutrients Such as carbohydrate, protein, fat, vitamins, and minerals. These are vital for maintaining bodily functions, supporting growth and repair, and preventing nutrient deficiencies that can lead to ill health.

Supports energy levels By providing the right mix of macronutrients (carbohydrate, protein, and fat), a balanced diet fuels your body with the energy it needs for daily activities (including workouts!). It helps maintain stable energy levels, preventing fatigue and enhancing physical and mental performance.

Promotes healthy weight management Eating in a balanced way helps regulate appetite and blood glucose levels, which in turn supports us to eat in tune with our bodies and maintain a healthy weight.

Reduces the risk of chronic diseases A diet rich in fruits, vegetables, whole grains, lean proteins, and healthy fats can lower the risk of chronic diseases such as heart disease, type 2 diabetes, and certain cancers. Nutrients and phytochemicals, for example, antioxidants, protect against inflammation and other factors that can contribute to these conditions.

Supports immune function Proper nutrition is key to a strong immune system. It provides the nutrients needed to fight off infections and illnesses, helping you stay healthy and recover more quickly when sick.

Supports mental health and mood The foods you eat can affect your mood and mental well-being. A diet that includes omega-3 fatty acids, vitamins, and minerals supports brain function, and also helps to protect against depression and cognitive decline.

Promotes hormone balance Hormones regulate many of the body's processes, including metabolism and mood. A balanced diet provides the nutrients necessary for hormone production and regulation, ensuring that these processes run smoothly.

Ensures long-term health Consistently eating a balanced diet maintains bodily functions, preventing nutrient deficiencies, and reduces the risk of age-related diseases. It helps your brain, heart, muscles, and bones to stay healthier. This in turn lets you lead a longer, happier life.

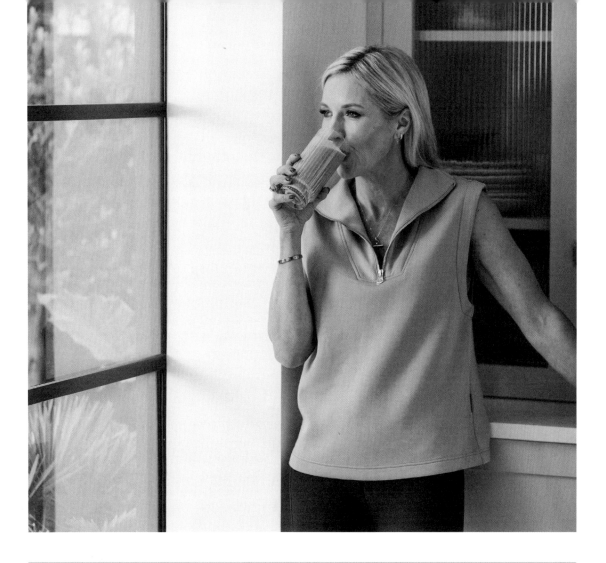

MY GOLDEN NUTRITION FUNDAMENTALS

- Eating regularly helps the body to function well and keeps our food decisions more proactive and nourishing.
- Try to cook your meals from scratch whenever possible.
- Make sure each of your meals checks off a source of carb, a source of protein, and a source of fiber.
- Include whole-grain carbs 2–3 times a day if you can, e.g., oats, brown rice or popcorn!

- Include plenty of plant-based diversity in your day. This is achievable even when your meals are based on animal proteins.
- There are no rules on when you should eat certain foods. If you prefer to have a bigger plate at lunch and a smaller bite in the evening, or vice versa, then that's fine. You may also feel more comfortable eating a substantial breakfast after you've trained. Let your own body guide you here as we're all different.

SLEEPING WELL

Sleep is our superpower! I cannot emphasize enough the importance of a good night's sleep for both our physical and mental well-being.

Many women who have always had great sleep patterns really struggle at this midlife stage, myself included. Insomnia is a symptom of menopause and affects so many of us. With the shift in hormones (particularly the levels of estrogen and progesterone), we can suffer from poor sleep routines. Alongside increased anxiety, hot flashes, and painful joints, a disturbed night can dramatically affect our mood and energy levels (as well as our exercise and food choices) the following day.

Sleep is an essential function; our bodies need it to rest, recharge, and repair. Sleep keeps our bodies strong, supports immunity, and prevents injury. It keeps us fit and healthy.

Research suggests that adults aged 26–64 need 7–9 hours of sleep per night and those over 65 need 7–8 hours. For many of us, this might not always be achievable—but it's something we can all aim for. We go through sleep cycles of 90–120 minutes, which consist of lighter and deeper sleep. Throughout these stages, your body has a chance to recharge and refresh.

WHAT IF WE DON'T GET ENOUGH SLEEP?

An insufficient amount of sleep over a prolonged period can lead to a higher risk of certain medical conditions, including high blood pressure, heart disease, stroke, and poor mental health. With inadequate sleep, it has been proven that our calorie intake the following day is increased and in turn it triggers the stress hormone cortisol, which can cause our bodies to store fat. Lack of sleep also affects our focus, attention, reaction time, and cognition.

Did you know?

Lack of sleep can interfere with so many of our daily functions, from our focus, stress levels, and immunity, as well as contributing to many health problems, such as high blood pressure, heart disease, and depression.

I also want to draw attention to the relationship between sleep and exercise. Exercise can really help your sleep. Research has shown that it not only helps you fall asleep faster but also improves your sleep quality. A good sleep will also have a huge impact on muscle recovery and repair. If you're strength training, running, or doing anything that challenges your muscles, then you're going to need your rest. As blood pressure and the heart rate drop after exercising and breathing becomes deeper and slower, the brain is fully resting, allowing more blood to reach your muscles. This delivers extra oxygen and nutrients to promote healing and growth. Remember too that exercise is a great stress reliever, so you may find you are less anxious at bedtime if you have moved that day.

TIPS TO IMPROVE YOUR SLEEP

- **Exercise during the day,** but not too close to bedtime, so your body has the chance to wind down.
- **Establish a realistic bedtime** and stick to the same routine as much as you can.
- **Avoid heavy meals** within a couple of hours of bedtime.
- **Jot down any worries** you may have and set them aside for tomorrow.
- **Practice calm activities** prior to bedtime, such as a relaxing bath or yoga.
- **Keep the lights low** if you can in the bedroom.
- **Think about a screen ban** before bed and maybe even in the bedroom.
- **Reduce your caffeine intake** in the afternoon.
- **Expose yourself to sunlight** when you wake up to help produce melatonin.
- **Take magnesium and ashwagandha supplements** for better sleep, reduced anxiety, and to promote muscle recovery. Not only do they help you fall asleep, but they also promote more restorative sleep. I make sure I get plenty through my diet, too, via dark leafy greens, nuts, and seeds, and also dark chocolate.

A POSITIVE MINDSET

The changes in our hormones during midlife, especially during menopause, can significantly impact our health.

Symptoms of anxiety, stress, loss of self-esteem, anger, and even depression affect so many women during this time. Joint pains (with the loss of estrogen), weight gain (often around the middle), migraines, and many other side effects of menopause can contribute to a reluctance to exercise. Often our own well-being and health needs are put to one side while caring for teenagers and elderly parents, alongside work and financial pressures.

Do you remember that I said at the start of this section that the four lifestyle pillars are interlinked? It's important to remember the (often vicious) cycle that can affect our mood. We have a bad night's sleep, this then makes us more lethargic and less inclined to want to exercise. The longer you avoid exercise, the less energized you feel, you make poor food choices, and feel low, etc. Once you can recognize the factors that are causing these feelings and break them down individually, you can start to find ways to make small changes,

which will lead to more positive experiences. It's important to remember that no one is perfect and change takes time.

YOU'LL NEVER REGRET A WORKOUT!

It has been proven that exercise can be particularly beneficial for our mental health. As little as half an hour of movement every day can give us a huge mood boost. Why is this? Exercise in any form reduces levels of the body's stress hormones such as epinephrine and cortisol. It stimulates the production of endorphins, a chemical found in our brains that works as the body's natural painkillers and mood elevator. Endorphins give a wonderful feeling of relaxation and are produced any time we exercise for long enough. Even if you don't always feel in the mood for it, a 30-minute workout can really change your mindset.

So set your alarm, lay your clothes out the night before, and try and move before the day takes over. Motivation is usually the hardest

"I LAUGH, I SHOUT, AND I FEEL SO MUCH BETTER FOR CHALLENGING MYSELF. AND THE BEST BIT? I'M NOW SEEING THE RESULTS!"

part, so make things easy and go for a walk (see pages 42–43). Being outside in nature is a wonderful mood booster and if you include some hills you will also be getting a great cardio workout too! Catch up with a friend and schedule walks in your calendar.

By beginning an exercise regime, you will start to notice how amazing endorphins make you feel. As these habits become established, you will begin to notice changes to your body, metabolism, heart health, and overall attitude, countering stress and relieving feelings of depression or anxiety.

A LITTLE CAN GO A LONG WAY

It doesn't need to be hours; even bite-sized chunks of exercise in your day all add up and really help. There are lots of ways to make exercise part of your day at home too—doing squats while the coffee brews, doing push-ups when you have a little downtime, and climbing stairs.

I particularly love my one weekly HIIT class for reducing stress levels and improving my mood. You will find HIIT workouts in the plan here too! However, it has been proven that too much high impact exercise can raise our cortisol levels, so I would recommend limiting these to once or twice a week (see pages 38–39).

If you're after something a little slower, stretching your muscles and completing exercises such as yoga will help to focus on posture and breathing, as will meditation, clearing the mind and reducing any anxiety that has built up. As the body feels more relaxed, it will in turn send mirroring signals to the mind to calm any mental tension. Moving your body will also help you sleep better (pages 26–27), allowing for both the body and mind to recharge and, in turn, support immunity and relieve anxiety.

SIX WEEKS TO A **STRONGER YOU**

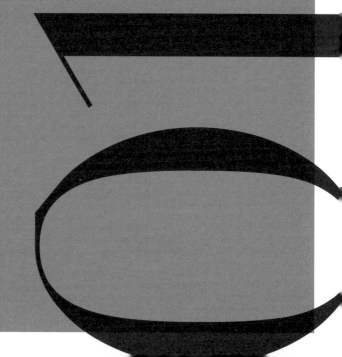

WHERE DO I BEGIN?

Beginning a new exercise program can be both exciting and challenging and often the hardest part is just getting started. I hope this book will inspire and motivate you to take this step.

I've known people who had barely exercised before and now cannot visualize their day without exercise. So how did they get there? Here are some top tips if you are feeling overwhelmed about taking the first step:

- **Set clear goals** Define your goals for strength training. Whether you want to increase muscle mass, improve overall strength, or enhance specific aspects of your fitness, having clear goals will help to guide your training program. Break down your goals into manageable weekly targets and celebrate each week's successes.

- **Schedule your workouts** Put the workouts in your calendar and block out that time in advance. Scheduling helps turn workouts into a regular part of your routine and helps you stick to your plan.

- **Plan with a friend** Tackling the six-week plan with a friend can increase motivation, making the process more enjoyable and fun.

- **Fuel yourself** Maintain a healthy, balanced diet rich in protein to support your workouts.

- **Learn the basics** Familiarize yourself with the basic strength-training concepts, such as sets, repetitions, and different types of exercises (see page 49 for more details). Understanding these fundamentals will make it easier to follow the workout routines.

- **Start with body-weight compound exercises** If you're new to strength training, begin with exercises without weights to build a foundation. Squats (see page 54), lunges (see page 65), push-ups (see page 74), and planks (see page 75) are excellent body-weight compound exercises that engage multiple muscle groups. The first two weeks in the plan are bodyweight-only: beginning slowly will allow you to avoid injuries and burnout, while getting started too quickly can be difficult and reduce motivation.

- **Understand proper form** Focus on correct technique and practicing proper form for each exercise. This is crucial to preventing injuries, ensuring that you're targeting the intended muscle groups and your body is in the correct position. A few good-quality reps are much better than lots of reps with poor form. I have included descriptions of all the exercises, as well as tips.

- **Practice progressive overload** This is where you gradually increase the resistance or intensity of your workouts over time to continue building strength. You can increase the weights and repetitions as you become stronger. The key is to build up slowly to avoid injury.

- **Warm up and cool down** Always start your strength training sessions with a warm-up to prepare your muscles and joints for exercise. Include dynamic stretches (where you are moving the muscles you are about to work, see pages 50–51). Afterward, cool down with static stretches to improve flexibility and aid recovery.

- **Listen to your body** Pay attention to how your body responds to strength training. If you experience pain (other than normal muscle soreness), modify your routine by reducing your weights or returning to body weight only. Seek advice if necessary.

- **Include rest days** Muscles need time to recover and grow stronger. Include rest days to allow your body to recuperate. Overtraining can lead to fatigue and an increased risk of injury so prioritize sleep and rest days to allow your muscles to repair. See pages 44–45 for more information about rest days.

- **Write it down** Document your daily activities to stay consistent. If you miss a session, don't stress—start again the next day.

Progress takes time, so be patient and stay committed. The workouts in this book are structured to help you build up slowly and increase your strength as you progress through the weeks. Celebrate your achievements and don't be afraid to adjust things as needed.

WHY
SIX WEEKS?

Significant changes will vary from person to person, as we all have different baseline levels of fitness. Six weeks provides a solid timeline to see initial results, both physically and mentally.

I have written a six-week exercise program for you because it is an ideal time frame for several different reasons. First, six weeks is the perfect period to begin to build muscle and increase your endurance. It typically takes 21 days to form a habit, and, so, six weeks will guarantee that you are well beyond this threshold, helping to make exercise a regular part of your lifestyle. By focusing on the right training program, with the correct rest and recovery, paired with a healthy diet, you will start to see those results that you've worked so hard for.

This defined timeline will also help you feel energized and maintain your focus and commitment, keeping you motivated on days when you are feeling distracted or tired. Although individual results will vary (and obviously depend on your starting level of fitness), six

weeks is enough time to observe improvements in strength, endurance, and overall fitness. As each week passes, I have gradually increased the intensity of the exercises to ensure continuous improvement. You will not only see tangible results, but will also have a sense of accomplishment, which will motivate you to continue on this journey, well beyond the initial six weeks.

"EVERY DAY I LOOK FORWARD TO GETTING UP AND DOING THE NEXT CLASS."

TIMELINE FOR SEEING RESULTS

2 WEEKS

- You may notice that your mood and energy levels have improved. Exercise releases endorphins, natural chemicals in the body that enhance mood and reduce anxiety.
- You are likely to find that your form and technique improve as your body adjusts to the exercises, making the movements feel more controlled.
- Your muscles may not tire as quickly as they did initially, allowing you to complete your sets with less fatigue.
- Seeing these small improvements will hopefully boost your motivation and confidence, encouraging you to stick with the program.

4–6 WEEKS

- You may start noticing a slight increase in muscle definition.
- You'll start to feel stronger and may be able to lift heavier weights or perform more repetitions than when you started.
- You may see an improvement in your posture, feeling taller and more confident!

- You might also notice that your body recovers more quickly from workouts, a sign that your muscles and cardiovascular system are adapting to your new routine.
- You may have better endurance, exercising for longer periods of time without getting tired.

BEYOND 6 WEEKS—once you have completed the program, there are so many ways to continue your progress in terms of strength, endurance, and overall fitness levels.

- After six weeks, your muscle size increases as the muscles continue to grow and strengthen. You can lift heavier weights and explore more challenging exercises, building on those in the final two weeks of the plan.
- Your body continues to get stronger: this strength helps with functional training, helping to make everyday tasks easier and more efficient.
- You are likely to see improvement in balance and coordination.
- Consistent strength training, especially when combined with a balanced diet, means that you are likely to see a reduction in your body fat percentage.
- After more than six weeks, strength training will become a regular part of your lifestyle, something you're committed to for the long-term. A habit that you enjoy!

WHAT IS FUNCTIONAL TRAINING?

An essential part of staying stronger for longer, functional training looks at our daily movement patterns and challenges our balance and coordination.

You will hear me talk about compound moves and functional training a lot in my workouts, and I thought it would be good to explain why they are so key to my midlife fitness programs. I have ensured that there are many examples of these movements in your six-week plan.

COMPOUND EXERCISES

Compound exercises are those that use more than one muscle group at a time: for example, when we squat down to lift something up and then reach to put it away or if we rotate to one side as we get out of a car. The term functional training, as it is known, can be a little confusing, since you would assume that all training has some functional benefit. This is true, but we are specifically talking about exercises that mimic these movement patterns we perform in everyday life.

For example, we sit down and stand up from a chair and then maybe we twist or turn at the top of the movement, or we get out of bed, or pick up groceries. These are actions we do all the time, but we don't often perform specific exercises to strengthen us for these movements. We have fallen into a trap of training like athletes for performance, rather than training for everyday movements.

FUNCTIONAL FITNESS

Functional exercises are key to preventing injury, trips, and falls and they generally enhance day-to-day living, especially as we get older. Did you know that more people get injured doing everyday activities (for example, lifting something heavy incorrectly), than they do working out in the gym? So, even though you may be strong at lifting weights in your exercise class or a great runner, it might not actually help you to move the lawn mower or pick up toddlers. Functional exercises and compound moves are essential for longevity!

Examples of these, which you will find in my workouts, are a squat and press (see page 87) or a renegade row (see page 87), or a deadlift into an upright row (see page 124). Ensure the weights you are using suit both parts of the movement and do not compromise your form. I always stress the importance of a strong core and which exercises that will help achieve this. Be mindful of posture, correct alignment, and the muscles you are working in each exercise at all times.

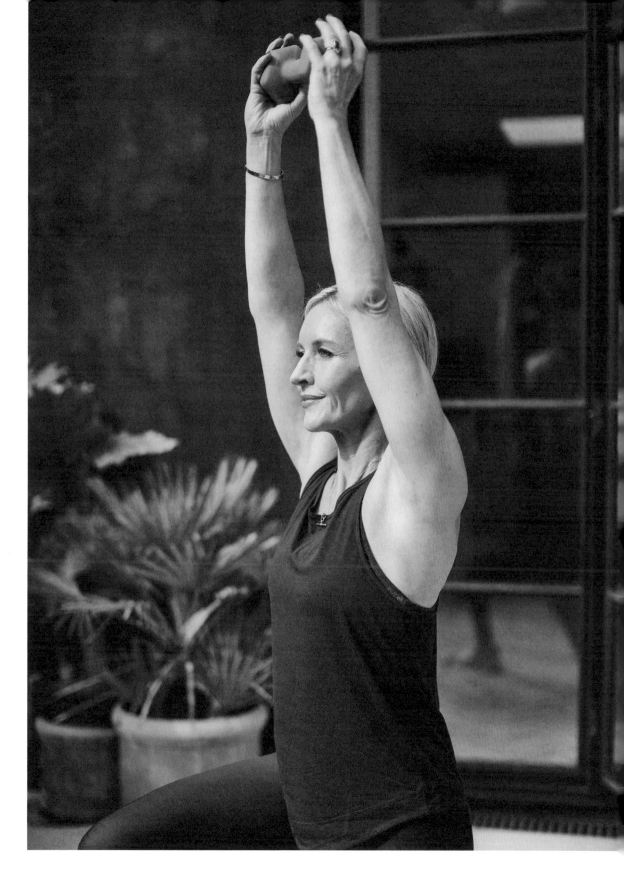

STRENGTH TRAINING VS CARDIO

I am regularly asked, "Strength or Cardio? Which is better?"
Before we answer this, let's clarify what I mean by each one:

CARDIO Activities that raise the heart rate, such as HIIT, running, walking, cycling, swimming, and hiking.

STRENGTH TRAINING Anything that involves working against resistance to build strength, for example, using weights or bands (such as the workouts in this book).

The choice between strength and cardio training depends on your fitness goals and overall health objectives. Both types of exercise offer unique benefits and, ideally, a well-rounded fitness routine would incorporate elements of both. Here's a breakdown of the advantages of each:

THE BENEFITS OF STRENGTH TRAINING

- **Muscle building** Strength training is highly effective for building muscle. It helps increase lean muscle mass, which can boost your metabolism and aid in weight management, especially important during menopause and midlife.

- **Bone health** Strength exercises improve bone density, reducing the risk of osteoporosis, which is especially important as we age.

- **Functional strength** Compound exercises enhance overall physical strength, making daily activities easier and reducing the risk of injuries.

- **Metabolic benefits** Strength training contributes to improved insulin sensitivity and better management of blood sugar levels, leading to better metabolic health.

- **Mental health** Resistance training can improve your confidence and self-esteem, relieving stress and anxiety, as well as enhancing cognitive function.

- **Joint health and injury prevention** Strengthening the muscles around joints provides added support, reducing the risk of injuries and promoting joint health.

EXAMPLE OF MY WEEKLY ROUTINE

- **Monday** Strength training *(full body)*
- **Tuesday** Strength training *(upper body)*
- **Wednesday** Strength training *(lower body)*
- **Thursday** Cardio: walk
- **Friday** Strength training/Cardio *(full body HIIT)*
- **Saturday** Rest day or light walk/yoga
- **Sunday** Rest day or light walk

THE BENEFITS OF CARDIOVASCULAR TRAINING

- **Heart health** Cardio exercises like running, cycling, and swimming improve cardiovascular health by enhancing heart and lung function.

- **Weight loss** Cardio workouts are effective for burning calories and can contribute to weight loss or maintenance.

- **Stress reduction** Cardiovascular exercise releases endorphins, which help reduce stress and improve mood.

- **Endurance** Regular cardio training improves endurance and stamina, making it possible to engage in sustained physical activities for longer periods of time.

A BALANCED APPROACH

A fitness routine that includes both strength and cardio training is ideal. Here's how I structure my own routine and what I suggest for others:

- **Strength training** Four sessions per week

- **Cardio** One HIIT class. In my workouts I have a strength HIIT session, which actually combines both elements!

This approach incorporates both types of training to provide comprehensive health benefits for optimum fitness. Think about your individual goals and what you want to achieve. Everyone is different, with unique goals and fitness levels, so it's important to tailor your routine to what works best for you.

WHEN SHOULD I INCREASE MY WEIGHTS?

I often get asked what size weights people should be lifting and when to increase them. Knowing when to increase your weights is essential for continued progress, motivation, and results.

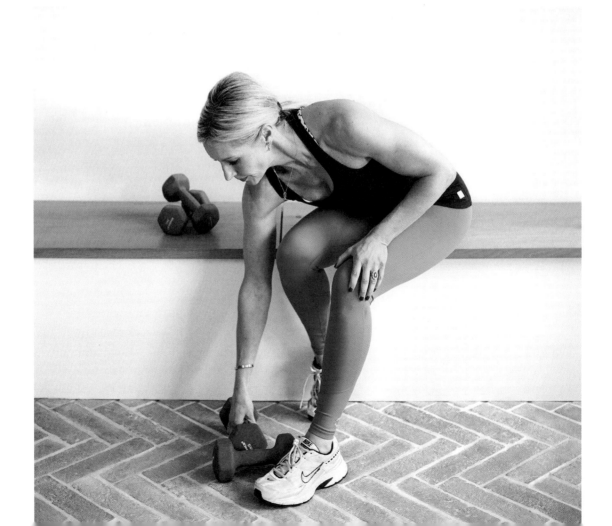

WHAT WEIGHTS SHOULD I START WITH?

If you are a beginner, I recommend that you start with 4lb (2kg) dumbbells and build up gradually. The key is to concentrate on technique and form before lifting heavy weights. Many of the workouts consist of higher reps with lighter weights. The reason for this is that I like to concentrate on endurance, as well as building strength for lean muscle, with correct technique always being the key focus. If possible, have a variety of weights to suit different muscle groups/exercises. For example, many people like to lift heavier weights for their lower body workouts and lighter ones for their upper body workouts.

HOW DO I KNOW IF I'M USING THE RIGHT WEIGHTS?

Here are some signs that it's time to adjust your weights:

- **Current weights feel too easy** If you find you can easily complete your sets and repetitions and it doesn't feel challenging any more, it is likely that you need to increase your weights. Your muscles need a sufficient stimulus to grow and adapt. Consider increasing your weights to maintain a challenging workout. Remember, it is key to build muscle in midlife.

- **Stalled progress** If you've noticed a plateau in your strength or muscle-building progress, increasing your weights can be beneficial. Your body adapts to the stress placed on it, so introducing new challenges is essential for continued improvement.

- **Lack of muscle soreness** While muscle soreness is *not* the only indicator of an effective workout, if you are no longer

Top tip

This is your journey— always use the weights that are right for *you*.

experiencing any soreness after your sessions it could mean that your muscles have adapted to your current routine. Gradually increasing your weights can help reintroduce that stimulus. You shouldn't be in constant pain post-exercise by any means, but knowing the difference between a challenging workout, which causes muscle fatigue, and an easy one, which doesn't, is key!

- **Changes in goals** If your fitness goals have evolved, for example, from endurance to strength, or from general fitness to hypertrophy (muscle growth), you may need to adjust your weights accordingly. Different goals often require different resistance levels.

- **Injury recovery** If you're returning to exercise after an injury or a break, it's advisable to start with lighter weights and gradually increase them as your strength and fitness levels improve. Listen to your body and progress at a pace that allows for proper recovery.

Remember that not every workout is about going heavy/heavier! There are lots of exercises that are about endurance—time under tension— without them involving a heavier weight. It's crucial to make gradual adjustments to avoid overloading your muscles and risking injury. If in doubt, start light and build up gradually. Aim for a progression that challenges you but allows you to maintain proper form during exercises.

WHY WALKING IS
SO UNDERRATED!

Simple, free, no special equipment needed, walking is one of the easiest ways to improve your health and fitness.

Walking is a great way to maintain your overall health. You will see in the workout program that I have recommended walking as part of your schedule and also as a great option for rest days. It has a whole list of benefits: it helps increase cardiovascular fitness, improve bone health, maintain a healthy weight, and it is also a huge mood booster. It also helps with our sleep patterns, which in turn improves immunity. Most importantly, being outside in nature has huge benefits alone. Not only for the production of vitamin D, but also for helping to reduce anxiety levels.

Unlike some other forms of exercise, walking is completely free, low impact, doesn't require any equipment, and you can get started right away, whatever your fitness level. It is a great way to build up muscle endurance, which helps with your sports activities too.

Try to go for a walk for at least 30 minutes every day. If you walk briskly, then this really is a great addition to your legs workout. If it's too difficult to walk for 30 minutes at once, try regular small bursts (10 minutes) three times per day and gradually build up to longer sessions. Go with a friend, or make your dog walks part of your weekly fitness regime.

Incorporating walking into your daily routine can be simple and enjoyable. By making small changes and gradually increasing the intensity, you can enhance your overall fitness, boost your mood, and enjoy the many benefits that walking has to offer.

HOW TO MAKE WALKING PART OF YOUR DAILY ROUTINE

1. **Take the stairs** Opt for the stairs instead of the elevator at work, at least part of the way. It's a simple way to add extra steps and build strength in your legs.

2. **Get off early** If you use public transportation, try to get off one stop earlier and walk the rest of the way to work or home. This small change can significantly increase your daily step count.

3. **Walk to the local stores** Whenever possible, walk instead of driving to nearby stores for last-minute groceries. This not only adds more steps, but also saves on fuel and reduces your carbon footprint!

4. **Keep a walking diary** Track how often you walk and how far. Keeping a diary can help you see your progress and ensure you stay motivated.

5. **Use a pedometer** A pedometer or a fitness tracker measures the number of steps you take. Monitoring your steps throughout the day and comparing them to other days or recommended amounts can motivate you to move more.

6. **Keep things varied** To prevent your body from getting used to the same routine, increase the intensity of your walks as your fitness level improves. Here's how:
   - **Walk up hills** Incorporate inclines into your route for a more challenging workout. Excellent for leg strength and cardio.
   - **Use hand weights or a backpack** Adding weight increases the intensity and helps build strength.
   - **Increase walking speed, distance, and time** Gradually include intervals walking at a faster pace in your routine. You can also walk a longer distance at a faster pace, before returning to a moderate pace, and extend the duration of your walks over time.

THE IMPORTANCE
OF REST DAYS

Throughout the exercise program, you will see sections marked as rest days. Why are these are so important?

I am a firm believer that the days you spend not training are just as important as the days you do! Personally, I *always* have two rest days per week, typically on the weekend when family life is busy. Rest days are critical to your fitness progression, especially when strength training—the days you are giving your body adequate recovery are the days you make gains in performance. The work you do in building strength, becoming fitter, or improving your stamina is done during a training session, but the gains are made in the rest and recovery. It allows your muscles a chance to repair, to make the changes you have asked of them, and will allow them to perform at their best during your next session.

During recovery, satellite cells repair the microscopic tears sustained during exercise. They replicate, mature, and fuse to the damaged muscle fibers. These in turn form a new muscle protein strand that increases the size and strength of the muscle to ensure it can keep up with future demand. This process is called hypertrophy.

Rest days are key to preventing injury and helping to avoid overtraining. If you expect your body to perform day after day without recovery time, it will start to break down—it's important to look after it!

Rest and recovery also allow your body to regulate its energy levels, resulting in a healthy, efficient metabolism that maximizes fat burning and total energy use. This replenishment of reserves is necessary to maintain energy levels, support upcoming exercise, and assist in effective weight loss (if this is your goal).

My advice is to train 3–4 times per week: for example, three or four strength sessions of 30 minutes, focusing on different muscle groups (see pages 38–39). On the other days, you can include some cardio if you wish, but walking as well as Pilates or yoga would give you a balanced training week. Allowing yourself those rest days will benefit you in the training days to come.

HOW CAN I PREVENT INJURIES?

When you feel like you're getting somewhere with your training, suddenly an injury rears its ugly head. Here are my top tips for staying in peak condition.

Don't run before you can walk!

Start gradually and build up slowly as your strength and fitness increase. Going in too hard, too fast is one of the leading causes of injury. It is great to hit the ground running and push yourself, but there is a balance!

Prioritize recovery

You can't expect results if you don't give your body the chance to recover, repair, and grow: if you train arms one day, focus on legs or core the next, or give yourself a rest day between challenging sessions. Use active recovery like walking, Pilates, yoga, or swimming to allow your muscles to recover and adapt.

Don't skip your warm-ups and cooldowns

The likelihood of getting injured increases dramatically when you neglect your warm-up and cooldown. This is why I include a warm-up of dynamic stretches and cooldown exercises in this book. I recommend that you spend 5–10 minutes at the beginning of every workout doing some dynamic stretches before the workout—these prepare the muscles for the workout to come, lubricate the joints, and improve blood circulation. Static stretches post-exercise will increase the range of motion in the joints and help muscles relax and ease tightness following your session. This will promote quicker recovery time. Try to dedicate 10 minutes to your cooldown too.

Focus on technique

This is key for weight training. Having good, correct form is vital to staying injury-free when strength training. The step-by-step images in the exercise section show the correct form for individual exercises.

THE EXERCISES

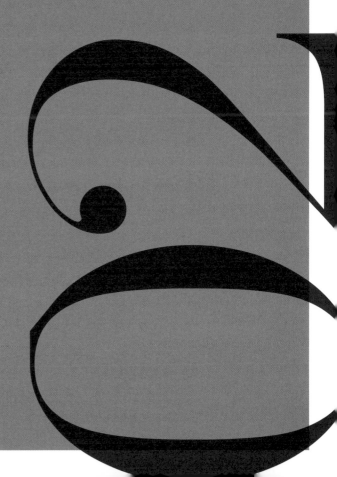

HOW TO DO
MY WORKOUTS

Short and sharp, my circuits are designed to fit in with your busy life. The guide here explains a little more about the exercises.

The workouts in this book incorporate the key principles of strength, functional, and HIIT training into 30-minute circuits (except the beginners' section, which are 20–25 minutes). Each circuit also includes both a warm-up and a cooldown (ideally 5–10 minutes for each). These circuits work different muscle groups and challenge your body.

There are four workouts per week over a six-week period. They are designed for all levels—from those who are new to exercise to people who have been working out for years. The weeks gradually build in intensity with the aim of helping you to get fitter and stronger as the program progresses.

WHAT YOU NEED

You need very little to get started, but here are a few suggestions that may be useful:

- A nonslip fitness mat.
- A short loop resistance band.
- 2 dumbbells (I suggest starting with 4lb (2kg) and increasing gradually as your strength improves). If you don't have dumbbells, don't worry; water bottles or cans of beans are just as good. As you progress and if budget allows,

I recommend having a heavier set of dumbbells for the lower body workouts and lighter weights for the upper body ones. The first two weeks of the program are designed to be done with just your body weight.

- Sneakers—for some of my classes, especially if there are high-impact exercises, wear sneakers for extra support.
- Water—always make sure you have plenty of water on hand and stay hydrated at all times! I also recommend rehydrating post-exercise to help recovery.

Scan the QR code below to access a guided Warm Up and Cool Down to welcome you to the 6-week programme and start you on your journey.

MY MOST USED EXERCISE TERMS

1 **Circuit** A set of exercises performed one after the other (also called interval training).

2 **Rep** This is short for repetition and is the number of times you perform an exercise before taking a rest. One rep is one completion of an exercise.

3 **Set** This is a group of exercises or repetitions performed in a row.

4 **Rest** The time spent resting between exercises or sets, allowing the muscles to recover.

5 **EMOM—Every Minute On The Minute** A form of interval training where you complete a certain number of reps within an allocated time. Once you have completed the exercises, you can rest for the remainder of the minute or perform a second exercise, depending on the program.

6 **AMRAP—As Many Rounds As Possible** A structured workout method where you perform as many reps or sets as possible within a fixed time frame back-to-back with no rest.

7 **Superset** Two exercises that are performed back-to-back with minimal rest. These can be exercises using opposing muscle groups or working the same muscles.

8 **Tabata** A high-intensity interval training workout that is designed to boost fitness in a short amount of time. Typically exercising for 20 seconds with a 10-second rest.

WARMUP

I recommend spending 5–10 minutes on these dynamic stretches before you start. Do 10–15 reps of each exercise.

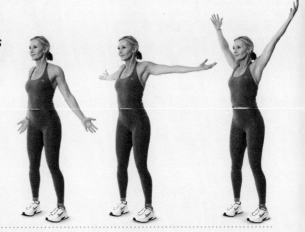

ARM CIRCLE

Standing tall, make big circles with the arms in both directions.

CHILD'S POSE

With knees wide, sink back onto your heels with your arms outstretched.

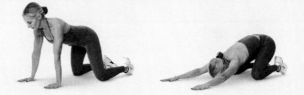

DOWNWARD FACING DOG

Start with your hands shoulder-width apart and shoulders above the wrists. Exhale as you lift your knees and reach your hips up and back. Bend each knee to stretch each leg in turn.

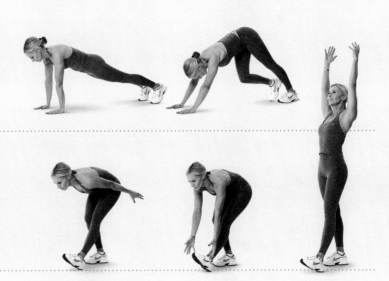

HAMSTRING SWEEP

On one heel, swipe low with the arms to stretch the hamstring and then open the chest at the top and reach high with the hands.

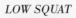

LOW SQUAT

With knees wide, bring the hips as low as possible, pushing the knees out with the elbows. Keep the chest lifted.

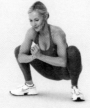

MARCH

Standing tall, bring
one knee up at a time,
shoulders back.

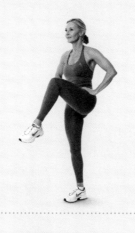

RUNNER'S LUNGE

In plank position, bring one foot
toward the hand. The other leg
can stay straight or you can drop
the knee to the mat. Lift the arm
and look up at the hand before
bringing it down inside the ankle
and switching sides.

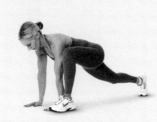

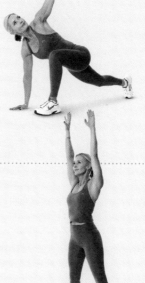

SQUAT TO REACH

Lower down into a wide
squat and then reach up
tall with the arms.

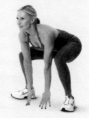

THREAD THE NEEDLE

With knees on the mat, raise one
arm, drop the shoulder to the mat,
and take the arm through and
underneath the body. Switch
sides. Try to keep the hips still.

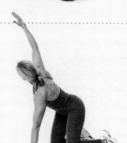

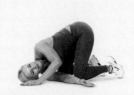

WALKOUT (OR INCHWORM)

Keeping your legs straight, walk
out your hands into a plank and
then back to the starting position.

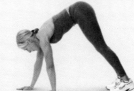

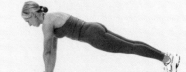

COOLDOWN

Make sure you spend 5–10 minutes on these static stretches to release muscle tension post-workout. Hold the positions for around 30 x secs each.

BACK STRETCH

Crossing the hands behind the knees, stretch the back.

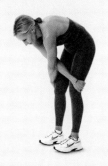

CHEST STRETCH

Place your hands in the small of the back and open the chest.

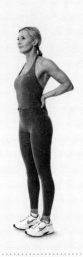

GLUTE STRETCH

Sitting up tall, tuck the knee into the opposite elbow and rotate the body to look over the shoulder.

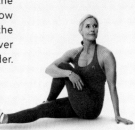

HIP FLEXOR STRETCH

On your knees, bring one foot forward, only coming as far forward as feels comfortable. Reach up with the arms.

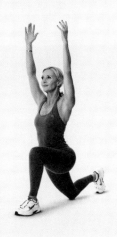

LOWER BACK STRETCH

Lying on your back, take the knees to one side and turn your head to look in the opposite direction.

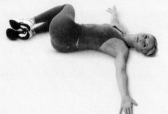

QUAD STRETCH

Standing tall, knees together, abs tight, take one leg at a time, bending at the knee with the foot toward the bottom to stretch the quad.

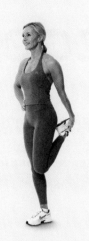

SHOULDER STRETCH

Take one arm across the body and hold. Repeat with the other arm.

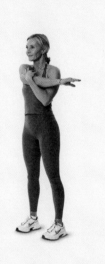

SIDE BEND

Reaching with your arms up, gently lean to the side, stretching the obliques as you lean from one side and then to the other.

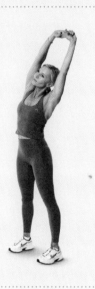

TRICEP STRETCH

Reach up tall with the arm and bend at the elbow with the hand behind the body. Gently stretch.

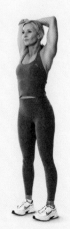

WEEK 01
MONDAY

Rest x 20 secs between exercises & repeat each circuit x 2 sets. Band or weight is optional here, but I recommend starting with no equipment.

CIRCUIT 1

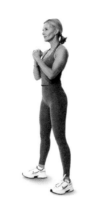
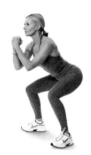

BODY-WEIGHT SQUATS

With all your weight in your heels, hips back, straight back, squat as if sitting into a chair, chest lifted, shoulders back. Come back up to standing and repeat.

x 10 reps

GLUTE KICKBACKS

From a tabletop position, with the core engaged, lift your leg behind you and squeeze glutes. (Don't take the leg too high.)

x 20 reps (x 10 each side)

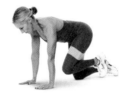
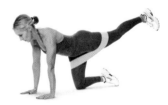

CIRCUIT 2

REVERSE LUNGES

(alternate legs)

With shoulders back and core engaged, step back to 90 degrees with one leg and power through the supporting heel to stand. Switch sides.

x 6 reps each side

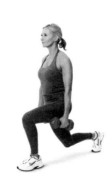
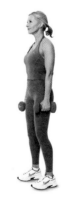

GLUTE BRIDGES

On your back with relaxed shoulders and neck, feet toward your bottom, tilt the pelvis toward you and drive up through the heels. Come down and repeat.

x 15 reps

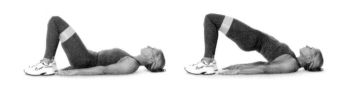

CIRCUIT 3

SPLIT SQUATS

Feet hip-width apart, shoulders back, core engaged, bend your knees so that they are at 90 degrees to the ground (or wherever feels comfortable), chest lifted, front knee behind the toe. Then come back to standing.

x 8 reps each side

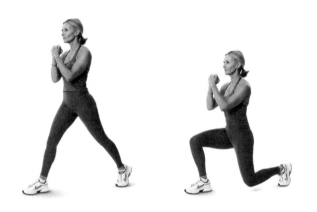

STANDING LEG RAISES

Keep the knee of the supporting leg slightly bent, stand upright and with foot flexed, slowly raise the leg straight up to the side (not too high) and lower back to standing.

x 10 reps each side

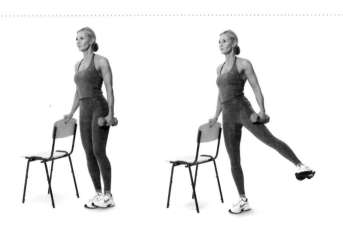

DONKEY KICKS

Start in a tabletop position, shoulders over wrists, abs tight. With foot flexed and knee bent, drive the foot to push away the ceiling. Don't twist the hips or go too high with the leg.

x 10 reps each side

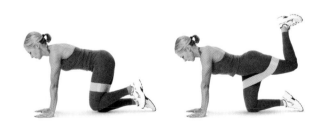

WEEK 01
TUESDAY

*Perform each exercise x 30 secs, rest x 20 secs between exercises
& repeat each circuit x 2 sets. Band or weight is optional here.*

CIRCUIT 1

BODY-WEIGHT SQUATS

With all your weight in your heels,
hips back, straight back, squat as
if sitting into a chair, chest lifted,
shoulders back.

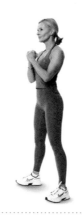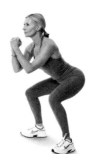

REVERSE LUNGES

(alternate legs)

With shoulders back and core
engaged, step back to 90 degrees
with one leg and power through
the supporting heel to stand.
Switch sides.

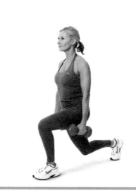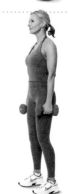

CIRCUIT 2

DEAD BUGS

On your back, head down or
off the mat, extend the opposite
arm and opposite leg slowly.
Switch sides. Keep the back on
the floor and core engaged
throughout. You can also do
this with light weights.

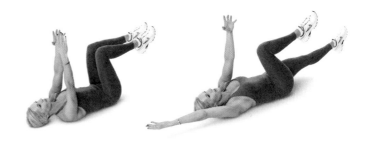

PLANK SHOULDER TAPS

(knees or toes)

Start shoulders over wrists, back straight, abs engaged, and head in line with spine. Slowly tap your hand to each shoulder in turn, trying to avoid movement through the hips. Squeeze the glutes.

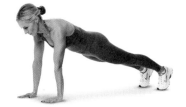 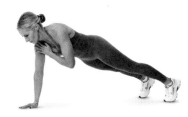

CIRCUIT 3

GLUTE KICKBACKS

From a tabletop position, with the core engaged, lift your leg behind you and squeeze glutes. (Don't take the leg too high.)

20 x secs each side

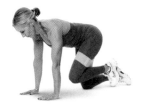 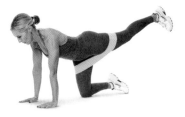

GLUTE BRIDGES

On your back with relaxed shoulders and neck, feet toward your bottom, tilt the pelvis toward you and drive up through the heels. Come down and repeat.

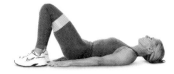 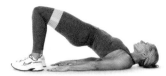

CIRCUIT 4

PUSH-UPS

With your hands wide on the mat, come forward in one movement (without dipping the head), back straight and elbows back. Try to keep core engaged and come up in one movement. Start against a wall or bench and progress to knees and then toes.

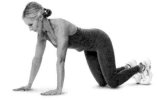 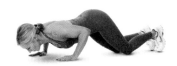

DORSAL RAISES

Lying face down, lift the head and shoulders off the mat in a very small movement. Do not come up too far and keep looking down.

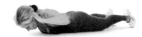 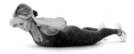

CIRCUIT 5

BICYCLE CRUNCHES

Without pulling on your head, bring opposite elbow to opposite knee, keeping your back down. Slowly extend the leg and switch sides. Go slowly to work the obliques without momentum.

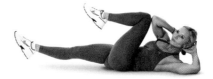

SLOW MOUNTAIN CLIMBERS

From a plank position, keep your hips down, back straight, core tight, shoulders over wrists, bring one knee into the chest and alternate. Do these at the right pace for you.

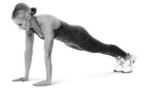 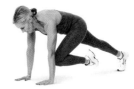

WEEK 01
WEDNESDAY

20 MINS
UPPER BODY
LIGHT WEIGHTS

Rest x 20 secs between exercises & repeat each circuit x 2 sets.

CIRCUIT 1

PUSH-UPS
(knees or toes)

With your hands wide on the mat, come forward in one movement (without dipping the head), back straight and elbows back. Try to keep core engaged and come up in one movement. Start against the wall or a bench and progress to knees and on to toe.

x 10 reps

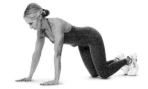
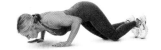

CHEST PRESSES

Keeping your elbows in your peripheral vision, imagine the letter "A" and press arms above chest (not the head), breathing out on the exertion.

x 10 reps

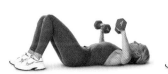
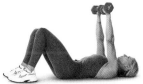

CIRCUIT 2

BENT-OVER ROWS

Hinge from the hips, with arms extended for full range of motion. Keep back straight and the head in line with the spine. Slowly bring arms back toward the pocket of your leggings. Core tight. Do not round spine.

x 10 reps

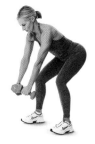
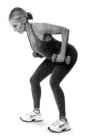

DORSAL RAISES

Lying face down, lift the head and shoulders off the mat in a very small movement. Do not come up too far and keep looking down.

x 10 reps

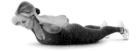

CIRCUIT 3

SHOULDER PRESSES

Knees soft, abs tight, keep elbows in line of vision. Slowly press the arms up and when lowered try to keep your elbows to 90 degrees.

x 10 reps

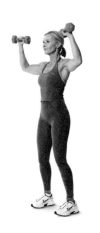
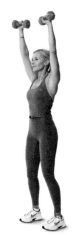

BICEP CURLS

Trying not to swing the arms, with your elbows locked into your side, slowly lift the weights and lower to the bottom and repeat.

x 10 reps

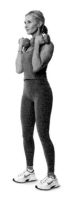
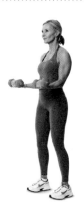

OVERHEAD TRICEP EXTENSIONS

(standing or kneeling)

Standing or kneeling with arms above your head, bend your arm back, keeping elbows close to ears. Slowly return to starting position. Don't lean back.

x 10 reps

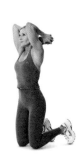
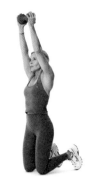

CIRCUIT 4

TOE TAPS

With your head off or down on the mat, bring your knees just above your hips and, alternating legs, slowly lower each toe to the mat, keeping your back down.

x 30 secs

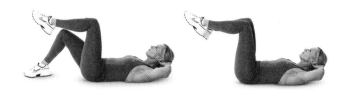

BIRD DOGS

In a tabletop position, move the opposite arm and leg to crunch in the middle and then extend both. Back stays straight and try not to twist through the hips. Do not raise the leg too high. Switch sides.

x 30 secs

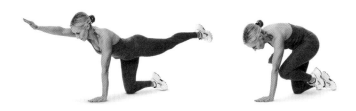

WEEK 01
FRIDAY

Rest x 20 secs between exercises, 10 reps per exercise & repeat the circuit x 2 sets.

CIRCUIT 1

DEAD BUGS

On your back, head down or off the mat, extend the opposite arm and opposite leg slowly. Switch sides. Keep the back on the floor and core engaged throughout. You can also do this with light weights.

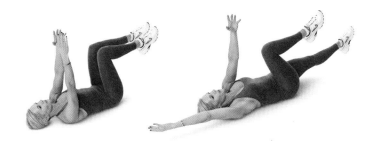

CRUNCHES

Bring your head and shoulders off the mat, back down, supporting the head without pulling on the neck. Keep a space between the chin and chest.

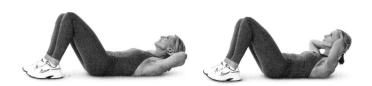

BICYCLE CRUNCHES

Without pulling on your head, bring opposite elbow to opposite knee, keeping your back down. Slowly extend with the leg and switch sides. Go slowly to work the obliques without momentum.

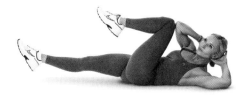

PLANK SHOULDER TAPS

(knees or toes)

Start shoulders over wrists, back straight, abs engaged, and head in line with spine. Slowly tap your hand to each shoulder in turn, trying to avoid movement through the hips. Squeeze the glutes.

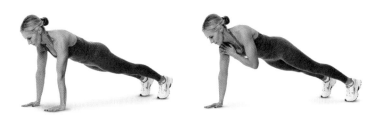

LEG EXTENSIONS

With your back down, only lower legs to where it feels comfortable and without your back coming off the floor.

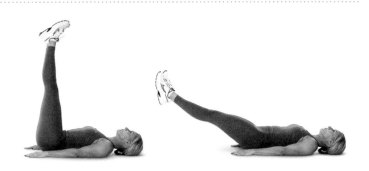

REVERSE CURLS

Keeping your head down, this is a small movement taking the hips off the mat. Try to relax your neck and shoulders.

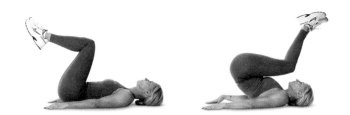

SLOW MOUNTAIN CLIMBERS

From a plank position, keep your hips down, back straight, core tight, shoulders over wrists, bring one knee into the chest and alternate. Do these at the right pace for you.

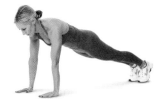 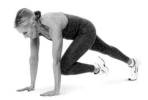

LOW PLANK KNEE TAPS

Keep in a straight line in a low plank position (no dipping with the head), then slowly lower each knee in turn.

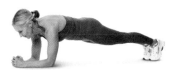 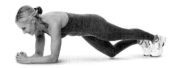

WEEK 02
MONDAY

20 MINS
FULL BODY
LIGHT WEIGHTS

Rest x 15 secs between exercises & repeat each circuit x 3 sets.

CIRCUIT 1

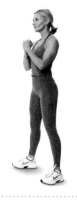
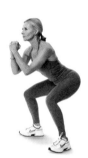

BODY-WEIGHT SQUATS

With all your weight in your heels, hips back, straight back, squat as if sitting into a chair, chest lifted, shoulders back.

x 10 reps

BENT-OVER ROWS

Hinge from the hips, with arms extended for full range of motion. Keep back straight and the head in line with the spine. Slowly bring arms back toward the pocket of your leggings. Core tight. Do not round spine.

x 12 reps

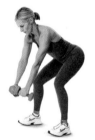
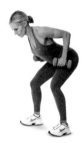

CIRCUIT 2

SHOULDER PRESSES

Knees soft, abs tight, keep elbows in line of vision. Slowly press the arms up and when lowered try to keep your elbows to 90 degrees.

x 10 reps

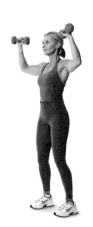
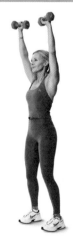

REVERSE LUNGES

(alternate legs)

With shoulders back and core engaged, step back to 90 degrees with the leg and power through the supporting heel to stand. Switch sides.

x 10 reps each side

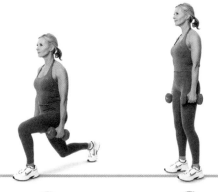

CIRCUIT 3

BICEP CURLS

Trying not to swing the arms, with your elbows locked into your side, slowly lift the weights and lower to the bottom and repeat.

x 15 reps

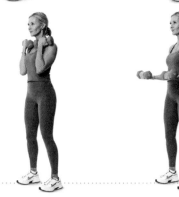

TRICEP KICKBACKS

In a tabletop position, slowly extend the arm to the line of your body without swinging. Avoid twisting the hips and keep the back straight, shoulders over wrists.

x 15 reps each side

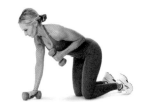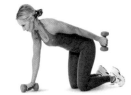

CHEST PRESSES

Keeping your elbows in your peripheral vision, imagine the letter "A" and press arms above chest (not the head), breathing out on the exertion.

x 15 reps

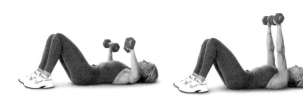

PLANK SHOULDER TAPS

(knees or toes)

Start shoulders over wrists, back straight, abs engaged, and head in line with spine. Slowly tap your hand to each shoulder in turn, trying to avoid movement through the hips. Squeeze the glutes.

x 10 reps

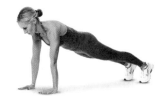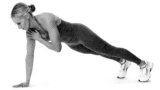

WEEK 02
TUESDAY

Rest x 15 secs between exercises & repeat each circuit x 2 sets.

CIRCUIT 1
CHEST

CHEST PRESSES

Keeping your elbows in your peripheral vision, imagine the letter "A" and press arms above chest (not the head), breathing out on the exertion.

x 10 reps

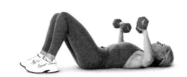
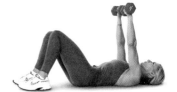

CHEST OPEN FLIES

Lie on your back with your head on the ground. Keep a slight bend to the elbows—open the arms, without resting on the mat, as you take them wide and then drive back to the starting position over the chest.

x 10 reps

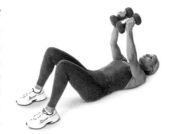
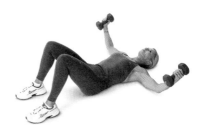

PUSH-UPS

With your hands wide on the mat, come forward in one movement (without dipping the head), back straight and elbows back. Try to keep core engaged and come up in one movement.

x 10 reps

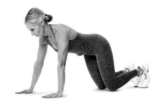
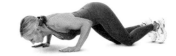

CIRCUIT 2
BACK

REVERSE FLIES

Hinge from the hips, back straight and core tight. Slowly open the arms to shoulder height and, without swinging, slowly lower, palms facing in.

x 10 reps

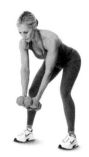
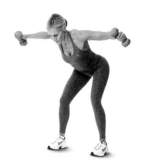

NARROW ROWS

Hinge at the hips, palms facing up. Use the full range of movement of the arms, back straight. Row the arms back, keeping the elbows close to your side. Squeeze at the top and keep your back straight throughout, head in line with your spine.

x 12 reps

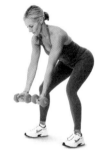
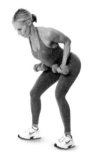

DORSAL RAISES

Lying face down, lift the head and shoulders off the mat in a very small movement. Do not come up too far and keep looking down.

x 12 reps

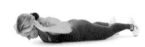
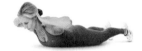

CIRCUIT 3
SHOULDERS

SHOULDER PRESSES

Knees soft, abs tight, keep elbows in line of vision. Slowly press the arms up, and when lowered try to keep your elbows to 90 degrees.

x 10 reps

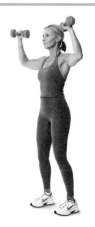
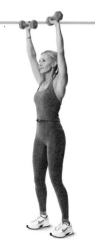

LATERAL RAISES

Without using momentum, knees soft, core engaged, slowly lift to shoulder height and lower. Bring the weights slowly down each time and try not to swing or lean back.

x 10 reps

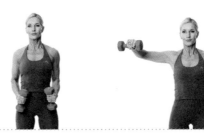

ALTERNATE FRONT RAISES

Slowly raise each arm alternately, without swinging or leaning back. Keep knees soft and shoulders back, chest lifted.

x 6 reps each side

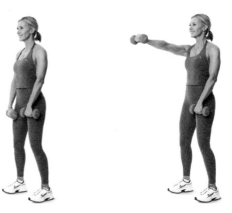

CIRCUIT 4
BICEPS & TRICEPS

TRICEP KICKBACKS

In a tabletop position, slowly extend the arm to the line of your body without swinging. Avoid twisting the hips and keep the back straight, shoulders over wrists.

x 10 reps each side

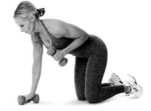
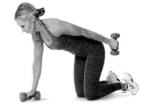

BICEP CURLS

Trying not to swing the arms, with your elbows locked into your side, slowly lift the weights and lower to the bottom and repeat.

x 12 reps

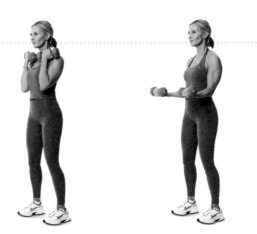

TRICEP DIPS

(on chair)

Keeping your back close to the surface of the chair, lower your body until your elbows are at 90 degrees, hands pointing forward.

x 10 reps

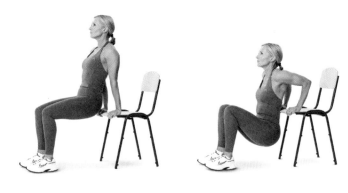

CIRCUIT 5
CORE

LOW PLANK KNEE TAPS

Keep in a straight line in a low plank position (no dipping with the head), then slowly lower each knee in turn.

x 10 reps

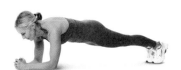
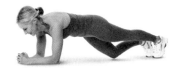

BIRD DOGS

In a tabletop position, move the opposite arm and leg to crunch in the middle and then extend both. Back stays straight and try not to twist through the hips. Do not raise the leg too high. Switch sides.

x 10 reps

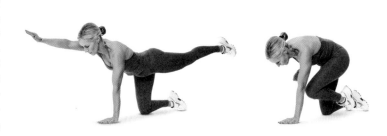

BICYCLE CRUNCHES

Without pulling on your head, bring opposite elbow to knee, keeping your back down. Slowly extend the leg and switch sides. Go slowly to work the obliques without momentum.

x 10 reps

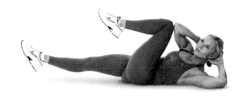

WEEK 02
WEDNESDAY

Rest x 15 secs between exercises & repeat each circuit x 3 sets.
Each exercise performed for x 30 secs. Band or weight is optional here.

CIRCUIT 1

CRAB WALKS

With or without a band, in a
semi-squat position, take three
strides across the mat and return,
keeping knees out and back straight.

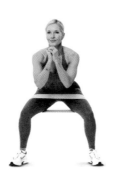
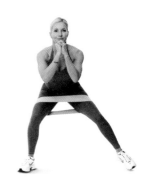

BODY-WEIGHT SQUATS

With all your weight in your heels,
hips back, straight back, squat as
if sitting into a chair, chest lifted,
shoulders back.

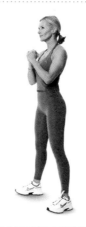
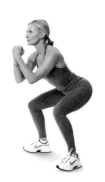

FIRE HYDRANTS

In a tabletop position without
twisting the hips, slowly raise one
knee to the side and slowly lower.

x 15 secs each side

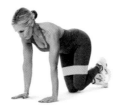
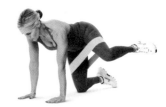

CIRCUIT 2

DONKEY KICKS

Start in a tabletop position, shoulders over wrists, abs tight. With foot flexed and knee bent, drive the foot to push away the ceiling. Don't twist the hips or go too high with the leg.

x 30 secs each side

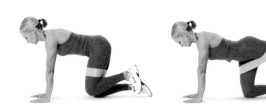

GLUTE KICKBACKS

From a tabletop position, with the core engaged, lift your leg behind you and squeeze glutes. (Don't take the leg too high.)

x 30 secs each side

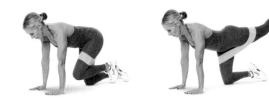

GLUTE BRIDGES

On your back with relaxed shoulders and neck, feet toward your bottom, tilt the pelvis toward you and drive up through the heels. Come down and repeat.

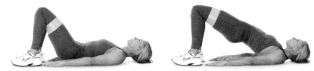

CIRCUIT 3

STANDING SIDE LEG RAISES

Keep the knee of the supporting leg slightly bent, stand upright, and with foot flexed slowly raise the leg straight up to the side and lower (not too high).

x 30 secs each side

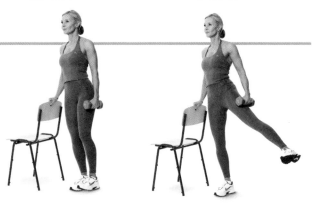

LATERAL LUNGES

Hips go back, chest lowers parallel to the thigh, other leg stays straight. Drive through the heel to push back to standing. Switch sides

x 30 secs each side

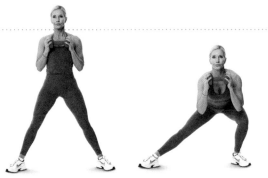

CLAMSHELLS

Lie on your side on the mat. Keep your feet together at the heel. Slowly raise the top knee, squeezing the glutes and slowly lower. Hips stay stacked and upper body lifted, abs engaged.

x 30 secs each side

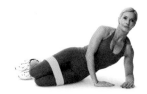
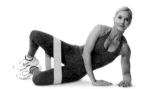

SPLIT SQUATS

Feet hip-width apart, shoulders back, core engaged, bend your knees so that they are 90 degrees to the ground (or wherever feels comfortable), chest lifted, front knee behind the toe. Then come back to standing.

x 30 secs each side

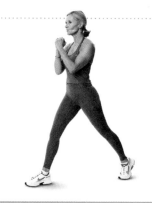
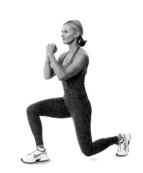

CIRCUIT 4
CORE

CRUNCHES

Bring your head and shoulders off the mat, back down, supporting the head without pulling on the neck. Keep a space between the chin and chest.

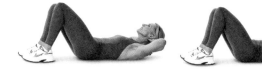

SLOW MOUNTAIN CLIMBERS

From a plank position, keep your hips down, back straight, core tight, shoulders over wrists, bring one knee into the chest and alternate. Do these at the right pace for you.

SLOW KNEE INTO ELBOW CRUNCHES

Standing with arms lifted, rotate at the hip bringing your elbow across to the opposite knee. Keep core engaged, back straight.

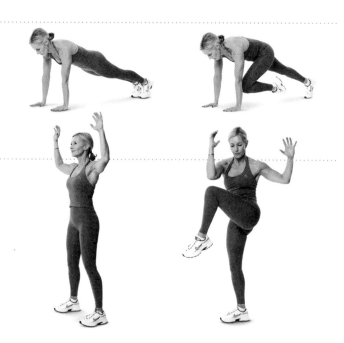

WEEK 02
FRIDAY

25 MINS
HIIT
BAND OR WEIGHT
OPTIONAL

Rest x 15 secs between exercises & repeat each circuit x 3 sets.
Each exercise performed for x 30 secs.

CIRCUIT 1

SHUTTLE RUNS

Take three strides across the mat, tapping down low at either end and bending knees while keeping the back straight.

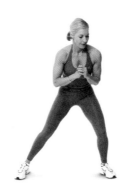
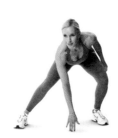

BODY-WEIGHT SQUATS

With all your weight in your heels, hips back, straight back, squat as if sitting into a chair, chest lifted, shoulders back.

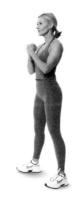
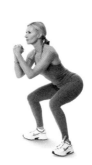

REVERSE LUNGES

(alternate legs)

With shoulders back and core engaged, step back to 90 degrees with the leg and power through the supporting heel to stand. Switch sides.

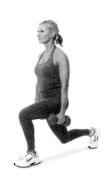
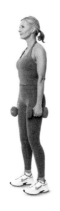

CIRCUIT 2

WALKOUTS

Keeping your legs straight, walk out your hands into a plank and then back to the starting position.

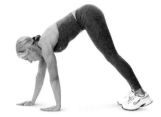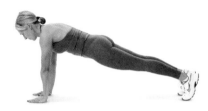

MOUNTAIN CLIMBERS

From a plank position, keep your hips down, back straight, core tight, shoulders over wrists, bring one knee into the chest and alternate. Do these at the right pace for you.

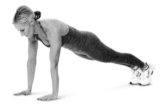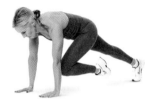

PUSH-UPS

With your hands wide on the mat, come forward in one movement (without dipping the head), back straight and elbows back. Try to keep core engaged and come up in one movement. Start against the wall or a bench and progress to knees and on to toes.

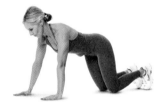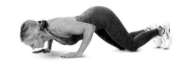

CIRCUIT 3

JABS

(no weights)

With core tight and knees soft, extend the arms, trying to keep the arms at shoulder level.

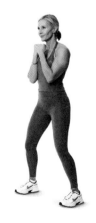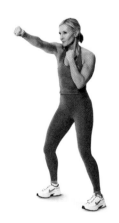

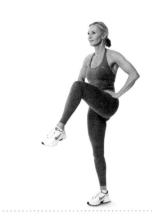

HIGH KNEES OR MARCHES ON THE SPOT

Standing tall, bring one knee up at a time, shoulders back.

PLANK HOLD

(low or high)

Shoulders over the wrists in either high or low plank position, bottom down, core tight. Glutes engaged. Back straight.

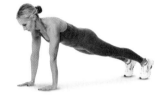
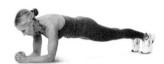

CIRCUIT 4

LATERAL LUNGES

Hips go back, chest lowers parallel to the thigh, other leg stays straight. Drive through the heel to push back to standing. Switch sides.

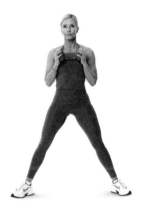
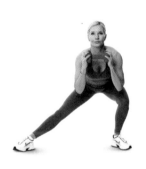

SQUAT INTO ELBOW CRUNCHES

With all your weight in your heels, hips back, straight back, squat as if sitting into a chair, chest lifted, shoulders back. As you come back up, rotate at the hip, bring your elbow to the opposite knee. Keep the core engaged and back straight.

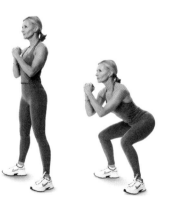
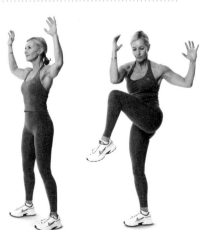

WEEK 03
MONDAY

Rest x 15 secs between exercises & repeat each circuit x 2 sets.

CIRCUIT 1
LEGS

GOBLET SQUATS

Sumo squat with the feet wider, toes out, and weight close to the chest. Hips back with your weight through the heels, drive back up.

x 12 reps

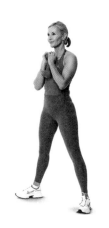
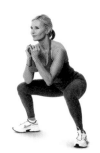

DEADLIFTS

With a soft bend to the knee, hinge from the hips, sending them back and keeping the back straight. As soon as the chest is parallel with the floor, drive up to stand. Try not to round through the spine or dip the head.

x 10 reps

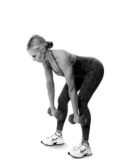
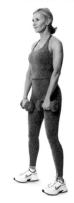

GOBLET SQUATS
WITH A PULSE

Sumo squat with the feet wider, toes out, and weight close to the chest. Hips back with weight through the heels; stay low for a pulse before driving back up.

x 12 reps

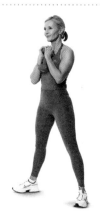
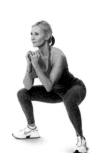

REVERSE LUNGES

With shoulders back and core engaged, step back to 90 degrees with one leg and power through the supporting heel to stand. Switch sides.

x 10 reps each side

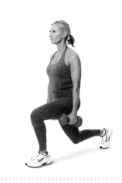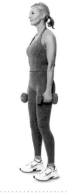

CURTSY LUNGES

Take one leg diagonally behind without twisting the front knee, keep upright with the body, and bend down as far with the back knee as is comfortable. Come back to stand and repeat.

x 8 reps each side

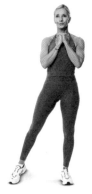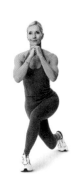

CIRCUIT 2
SHOULDERS

SHOULDER PRESS

Knees soft, abs tight, keep elbows in line of vision. Slowly press the arms up and when lowered try to keep your elbows to 90 degrees.

x 10 reps

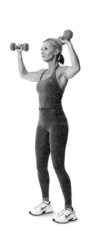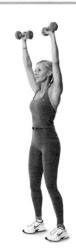

LATERAL RAISES

Without using momentum, knees soft, core engaged, slowly lift to shoulder height and lower. Bring the weights slowly down each time and try not to swing or lean back.

x 10 reps

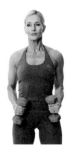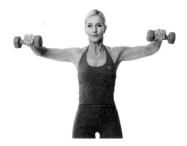

UPRIGHT ROWS

Standing tall with knees soft,
bring your elbows up
toward your chest.

x 10 reps

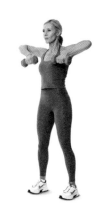
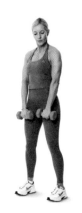

CIRCUIT 3
BICEPS & BACK

NARROW ROWS

Hinge at the hips, palms facing up.
Use the full range of movement of
the arms, back straight. Row the
arms, keeping the elbows close to
your side. Squeeze at the top and
keep your back straight throughout,
head in line with your spine.

x 12 reps

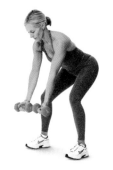
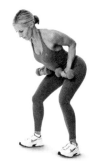

BICEP CURLS

Trying not to swing the arms, with
your elbows locked into your side,
slowly lift the weights and lower
to the bottom and repeat.

x 12 reps

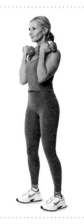
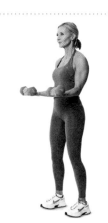

REVERSE FLIES

Hinge from the hips, back straight
and core tight. Slowly open the
arms to shoulder height and,
without swinging, slowly lower,
palms facing in.

x 10 reps

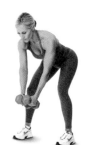
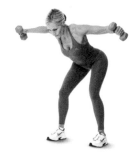

CIRCUIT 4
CHEST & TRICEPS

PUSH-UPS

With your hands wide on the mat, go down in one movement (without dipping the head), back straight and elbows back. Try to keep core engaged and come up in one movement. Start against the wall or a bench and progress to knees and on to toes.

x 10 reps

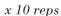
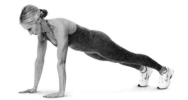
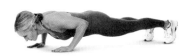

CHEST PRESSES

Keeping your elbows in your peripheral vision, imagine the letter "A" and press arms above chest (not the head), breathing out on the exertion.

x 12 reps

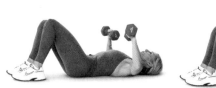
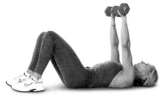

OVERHEAD TRICEP EXTENSIONS

Standing or kneeling with arms above your head, bend your arm back keeping elbows close to ears. Slowly return to starting position. Don't lean back.

x 12 reps

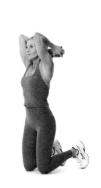
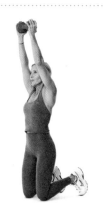

TRICEP KICKBACKS

In a tabletop position, slowly extend the arm to the line of your body without swinging. Avoid twisting the hips and keep the back straight, shoulders over wrists.

x 10 reps each side

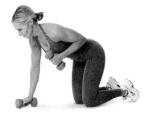
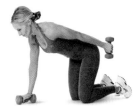

WEEK 03
TUESDAY

Rest x 15 secs between exercises.
Each exercise is performed x 12 reps.

SUPER SET

x 3 sets

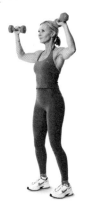
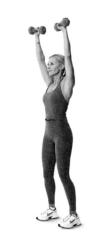

SHOULDER PRESSES

Knees soft, abs tight, keep elbows in line of vision. Slowly press the arms up and when lowered try to keep your elbows to 90 degrees.

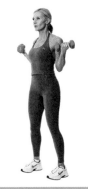
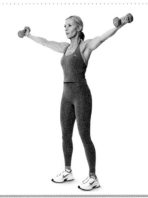

Y PRESSES

Using lighter weights or body weight, take your hands directly out to the sides at shoulder height and then draw the elbows back toward the body and slightly behind, squeezing the back muscles as you do so.

SUPER SET

x 3 sets

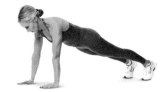
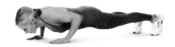

PUSH-UPS

With your hands wide on the mat, go down in one movement (without dipping the head), back straight and elbows back. Try to keep core engaged and come up in one movement. Start against the wall or a bench and progress to knees and on to toes.

CHEST PRESSES

Keeping your elbows in your peripheral vision, imagine the letter "A" and press arms above chest (not the head), breathing out on the exertion.

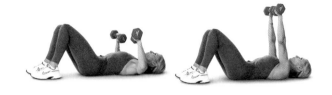

SUPER SET

x 3 sets

NARROW ROWS

Hinge at the hips, palms facing up. Use the full range of movement of the arms, back straight. Row the arms, keeping the elbows close to your side. Squeeze at the top and keep your back straight throughout, head in line with your spine.

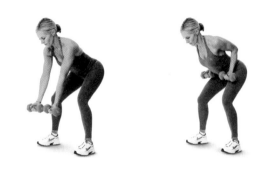

DORSAL RAISES

Lying face down, lift the head and shoulders off the mat in a very small movement. Do not come up too far and keep looking down.

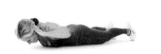
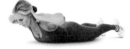

SUPER SET

x 2 sets

SKULL CRUSHERS

Lying down—using one weight or two—keep elbows tucked in as you take the weight behind the head. Bring back to starting position and repeat. Only the lower part of the arm moves.

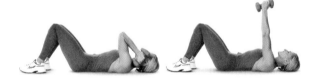

TRICEP DIPS

Keeping your back close to the surface of the chair, lower your body until your elbows are at 90 degrees, hands pointing forward, then come back up.

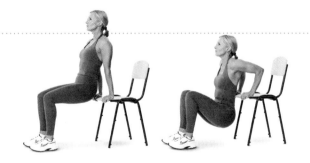

SUPER SET

x 2 sets

DEAD BUGS

On your back, head down or off the mat, extend the opposite arm and opposite leg slowly before returning to start position. Switch sides. Keep the back on the floor and core engaged throughout. You can also do this with light weights.

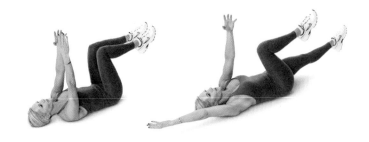

RUSSIAN TWISTS

Feet can stay down or come off the mat. Slowly turn from side to side without moving the knees. Keep abs tight throughout. Perform with or without weights.

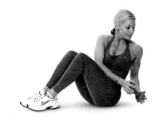 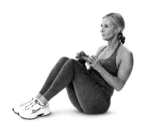

SUPER SET

x 2 sets

HIGH PLANK SHOULDER TAPS

Start shoulders over wrists, back straight, abs engaged, and head in line with spine. Slowly tap your hand across each shoulder in turn, trying to avoid movement through the hips. Squeeze the glutes.

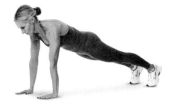 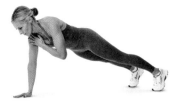

LOW PLANK KNEE TAPS

Keep in a straight line in a low plank position (no dipping with the head), then slowly lower each knee in turn.

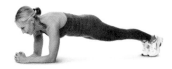 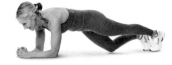

WEEK 03
WEDNESDAY

30 MINS
LOWER BODY
BODY WEIGHT/BAND

Rest x 15 secs between exercises & repeat each circuit x 2 sets.

CIRCUIT 1

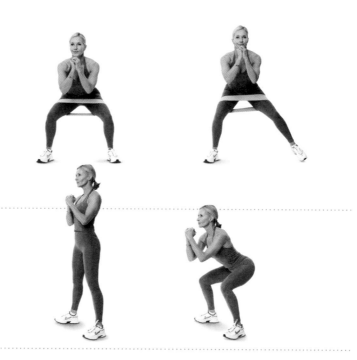

CRAB WALKS

With or without a band, in a semi-squat position, take three strides across the mat and return, keeping knees out and back straight.

x 10 reps

BODY-WEIGHT SQUATS

With all your weight in your heels, hips back, straight back, squat as if sitting into a chair, chest lifted, shoulders back.

x 10 reps

DONKEY KICKS

Start in a tabletop position, shoulders over wrists, abs tight. With foot flexed and knee bent, drive the foot to push away the ceiling. Don't twist the hips or go too high with the leg.

x 10 reps each side

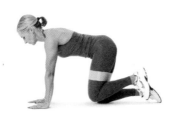
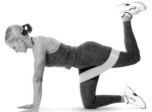

FIRE HYDRANTS

In a tabletop position without twisting the hips, slowly raise one knee to the side and slowly lower.

x 10 reps each side

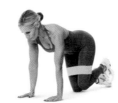
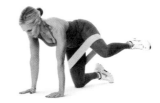

GLUTE BRIDGES

On your back with relaxed shoulders and neck, feet toward your bottom, tilt the pelvis toward you and drive up through the heels. Come down and repeat.

x 15 reps

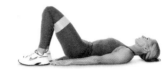
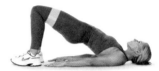

CIRCUIT 2

STANDING LEG RAISES

(each side)

Keep the knee of the supporting leg slightly bent, stand upright and with foot flexed slowly raise the leg straight up to the side (not too high) and lower back to standing.

x 10 reps each side

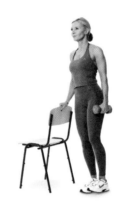
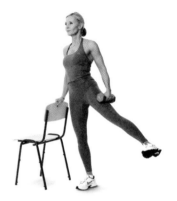

SQUATS WITH A PULSE

With all your weight in your heels, hips back, straight back, squat as if sitting into a chair, chest lifted, shoulders back. Stay low for a pulse before standing.

x 12 reps

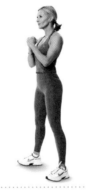
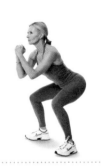

REVERSE LUNGES

(alternate legs)

With shoulders back and core engaged, step back to 90 degrees with one leg and power through the supporting heel to stand. Switch sides.

x 10 reps each side

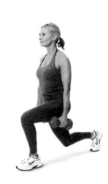
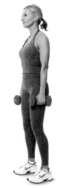

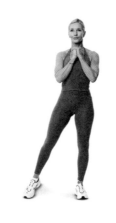
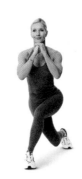

CURTSY LUNGES

(alternating sides)

Take one leg diagonally behind without twisting the front knee, keep upright with the body, and bend down as far with the back knee as is comfortable. Come back to stand and repeat.

x 12 reps

CIRCUIT 3

CLAMSHELLS

Lie on your side on the mat. Keep your feet together at the heel. Slowly raise the top knee, squeezing the glutes and slowly lower. Hips stay stacked and upper body lifted, abs engaged.

x 10 reps each side

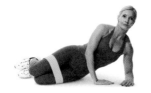
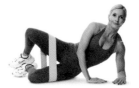

SIDE-LYING LEG RAISES

In a straight line with hips stacked, and lower leg bent, slowly raise the top leg with foot flexed and slowly lower. Keep the core engaged.

x 12 reps each side

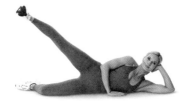

GLUTE KICKBACKS

From a tabletop position, with the core engaged, lift your leg behind you and squeeze glutes. (Don't take the leg too high.)

x 12 reps each side

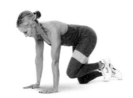
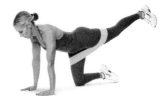

WALL SQUATS

With knees at 90 degrees and back against the wall, try not to let hands rest on the legs.

Hold x 30 secs

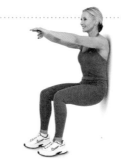

CIRCUIT 4
CORE

BIRD DOGS

In a tabletop position, move the opposite arm and leg to crunch in the middle and then extend both. Back stays straight and try not to twist through the hips. Do not raise the leg too high. Switch sides.

x 10 reps each side

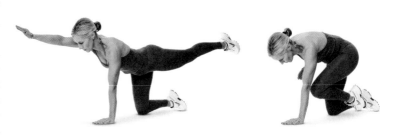

CRUNCHES

Bring your head and shoulders off the mat, back down, supporting the head without pulling on the neck. Keep a space between the chin and chest.

x 10 reps

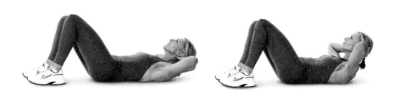

LEG EXTENSIONS

With your back down, only lower legs to where it feels comfortable and without your back coming off the floor.

x 10 reps

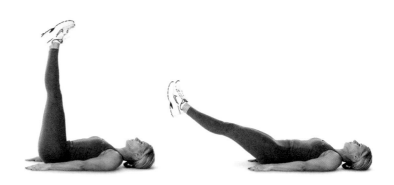

CROSS CLIMBERS

With shoulders over wrists and core engaged, bring each knee under the body toward the opposite elbow. Minimize movement through the hips and keep the back straight.

x 10 reps

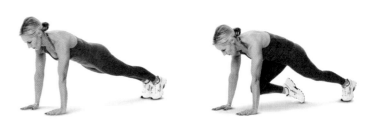

WEEK 03
FRIDAY

30 MINS
STRENGTH HIIT
BODY WEIGHT/WEIGHTS

Perform each exercise x 30 secs. Rest x 15 secs between exercises & repeat each circuit x 3 sets. Rest for 1 minute in between each circuit.

CIRCUIT 1

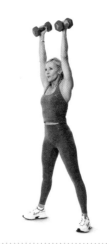

SQUAT AND PRESS

Lower into the squat position and as you come back to standing raise the arms into a shoulder press.

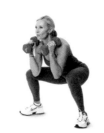

RENEGADE ROWS

(knees or toes)

In a plank position, avoid movement through the hips, drive the weight back close to your side (with elbows in) toward the back pocket of your leggings. Bottom down and straight back. You can start on your knees and progress to a plank.

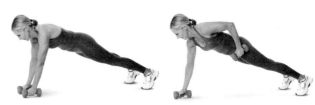

SHUTTLE RUNS

Take three strides across the mat, tapping down low at either end and bending knees while keeping the back straight.

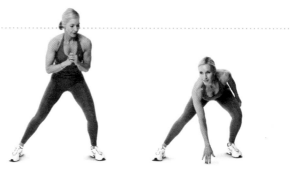

PLANK SHOULDER TAPS

Start shoulders over wrists, back straight, abs engaged, and head in line with spine. Slowly tap your hand to each shoulder in turn, trying to avoid movement through the hips. Squeeze the glutes.

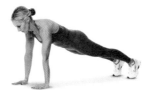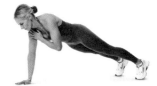

CIRCUIT 2

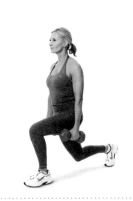
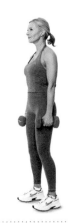

REVERSE LUNGES

(alternate legs)

With shoulders back and core engaged, step back to 90 degrees with one leg and power through the supporting heel to stand. Switch sides.

PUSH-UPS

With your hands wide on the mat, go down in one movement (without dipping the head), back straight and elbows back. Try to keep core engaged and come up in one movement. Start against the wall or a bench and progress to knees and on to toes.

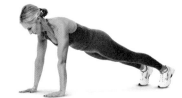
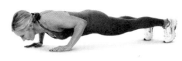

FAST JABS

With core tight and knees soft, extend the arms, trying to keep the arms/weights at shoulder level.

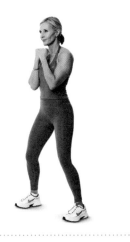
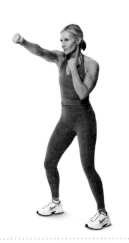

BICYCLE CRUNCHES

Without pulling on your head, bring opposite elbow to knee, keeping your back down. Slowly extend the leg and switch sides. Go slowly to work the obliques without momentum.

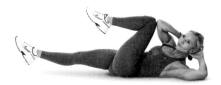

CIRCUIT 3

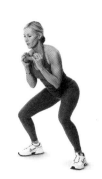
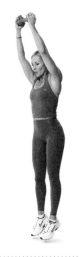

SQUAT JUMP AND PRESS

Start with a squat and when you get to the bottom of the squat, jump, bringing your legs together and press weight overhead. For a low-impact variation, take out the jump.

BICEP CURLS TO SHOULDER PRESS

Trying not to swing the arms, with your elbows locked into your side, slowly lift the weights into a bicep curl and then take the weights overhead into a shoulder press. Lower and repeat.

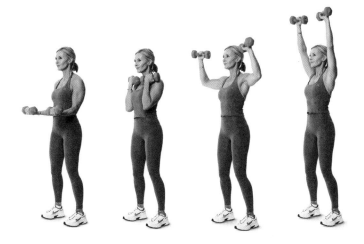

WALKOUTS

Keeping your legs straight, walk out your hands into a plank and then back to the starting position.

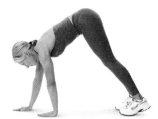
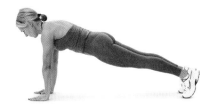

MOUNTAIN CLIMBERS

From a plank position, keep your hips down, back straight, core tight, shoulders over wrists, bring one knee into the chest and alternate. Do these at the right pace for you.

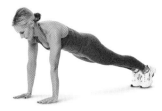
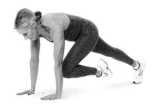

WEEK 04
MONDAY

Perform each exercise x 12 reps. Rest x 15 secs between exercises & repeat each circuit x 2 sets.

CIRCUIT 1

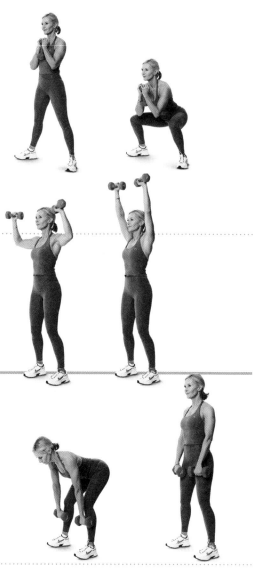

GOBLET SQUATS

Sumo squat with the feet wider, toes out, and weight close to the chest. Hips back with your weight through the heels, drive back up.

SHOULDER PRESSES

Knees soft, abs tight, keep elbows in line of vision. Slowly press the arms up and when lowered try to keep your elbows to 90 degrees.

CIRCUIT 2

DEADLIFTS

With a soft bend to the knee, hinge from the waist, sending the hips back, keeping the back straight. As soon as the chest is parallel with the floor, drive up to stand. Try not to round through the spine or dip the head.

BENT-OVER ROWS

Hinge from the hips, with arms extended for full range of motion. Keep back straight and the head in line with the spine. Slowly bring arms back toward the pocket of your leggings. Core tight. Do not round spine.

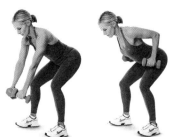

Y PRESSES

Using lighter weights or body weight, take your hands directly out to the sides at shoulder height and then draw the elbows back toward the body and slightly behind, squeezing the back muscles as you do so.

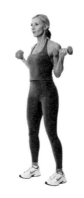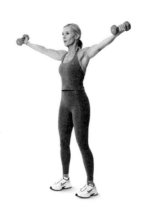

CIRCUIT 3

REVERSE LUNGES

(alternate legs)

With shoulders back and core engaged, step back to 90 degrees with one leg and power through the supporting heel to stand. Switch sides

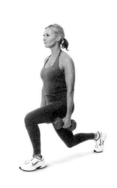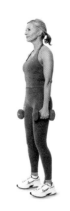

SPLIT SQUATS

Feet hip-width apart, shoulders back, core engaged, bend your knees so that they are 90 degrees to the ground (or wherever feels comfortable), chest lifted, front knee behind the toe. Come back to stand and repeat.

x 12 reps each side

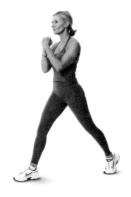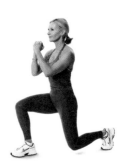

TRICEP KICKBACKS

In a tabletop position, slowly extend the arm to the line of your body without swinging. Avoid twisting the hips and keep the back straight, shoulders over wrists.

x 12 reps each side

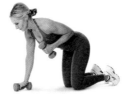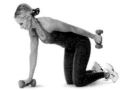

CIRCUIT 4

CHEST PRESSES

Keeping your elbows in your peripheral vision, imagine the letter "A" and press arms above chest (not the head), breathing out on the exertion.

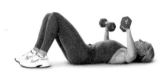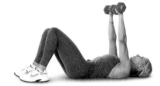

BENT KNEE JACKKNIVES

Keeping back down, crunch into a ball and slowly extend arms and legs (only to where it feels comfortable).

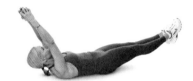

CIRCUIT 5

SQUAT AND PRESS

Lower into the squat position and as you come back to standing raise the arms into a shoulder press.

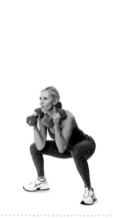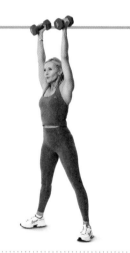

DEADLIFT INTO UPRIGHT ROWS

With a soft bend to the knee, hinge from the hips, sending them back, keeping the back straight. As soon as the chest is parallel with the floor, drive up to stand. Try not to round through the spine or dip the head. Standing tall with knees soft, bring your elbows up toward your chest.

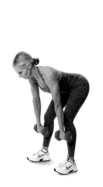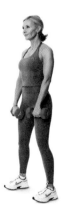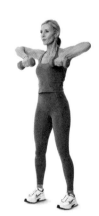

CIRCUIT 6
CORE

TOE TAPS

With your head off or down on the mat, bring your knees just above your hips and slowly lower each toe in turn to the mat. Ensure you keep your back down.

x 20 secs

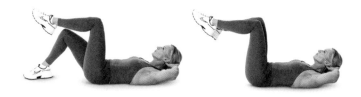

REVERSE CURLS

Keeping your head down, this is a small movement, taking the hips off the mat. Try to relax your neck and shoulders.

x 20 secs

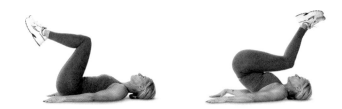

SIDE PLANK HOLD

With elbow directly under the shoulder, hold the position with core engaged and hips stacked (can be done on knees).

Hold x 20 secs each side

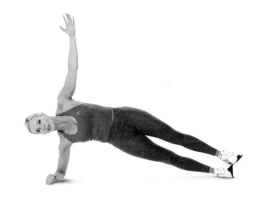

PLANK HOLD
(high or low)

Shoulders over the wrists in either high or low plank position, bottom down, core tight. Glutes engaged. Back straight.

Hold x 20 secs

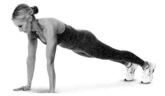
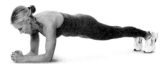

WEEK 04
TUESDAY

Rest x 15 secs between exercises & repeat each circuit x 3 sets.
Perform a shoulder press for 10 reps between each circuit.

CIRCUIT 1

CHEST PRESSES

Keeping your elbows in your peripheral vision, imagine the letter "A" and press arms above chest (not the head), breathing out on the exertion.

x 12 reps

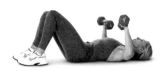 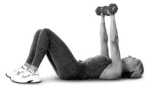

PUSH-UPS

With your hands wide on the mat, go down in one movement (without dipping the head), back straight and elbows back. Come over the hands and then push back to start through the heel of the hands. Try to keep core engaged and come up again in one movement. Start against the wall or a bench and progress to knees and on to toes.

x 12 reps

REPEAT THIS BETWEEN EACH CIRCUIT

SHOULDER PRESSES

Knees soft, abs tight, keep elbows in line of vision. Slowly press the arms up and when lowered try to keep your elbows to 90 degrees.

x 10 reps

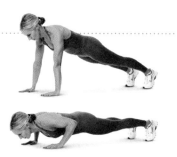

CIRCUIT 2

SKULL CRUSHERS

Lying down—using one weight or two— keep elbows tucked in as you take the weight behind the head. Bring back to starting position and repeat. Only the lower part of the arm moves.

x 10 reps

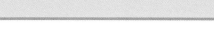
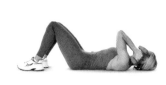
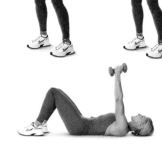

TRICEP KICKBACKS

In a tabletop position, slowly extend the arm to the line of your body without swinging. Avoid twisting the hips and keep the back straight, shoulders over wrists.

x 10 reps each side

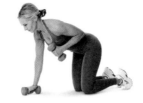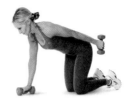

CIRCUIT 3

LATERAL RAISES

Without using momentum, knees soft, core engaged, slowly lift to shoulder height and lower. Bring the weights slowly down each time and try not to swing or lean back.

x 8 reps

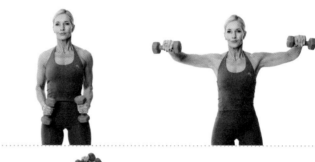

OPEN CHEST FLIES

Lie on your back with your head on the ground. Keep a slight bend to the elbows—open the arms, without resting on the mat as, you take them wide and then drive back to the starting position over the chest.

x 8 reps

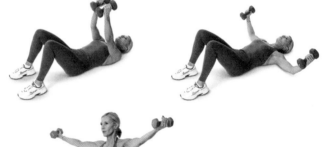

AIRPLANES

Using light or no weights, try to keep the arms at shoulder height and draw little circles in one direction and then the other.

x 8 reps each direction

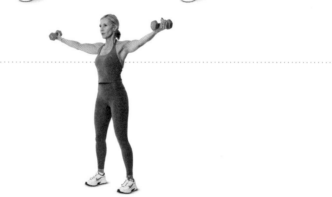

PLANK HOLD (high or low)

Shoulders over the wrists in either high or low plank position, bottom down, core tight. Glutes engaged. Back straight.

Hold x 1 min

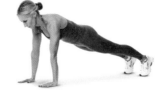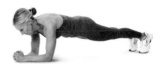

WEEK 04
WEDNESDAY

Rest x 15 secs between exercises & repeat each circuit x 2 sets. Perform x 10 squat jumps and press in between each circuit.

CIRCUIT 1

CRAB WALKS

With or without a band, in a semi-squat position, take three strides across the mat and return, keeping knees out and back straight.

x 30 secs

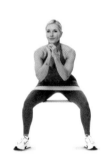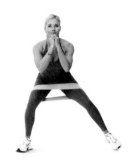

FIRE HYDRANTS

In a tabletop position without twisting the hips, slowly raise one knee to the side and slowly lower.

x 15 secs each side

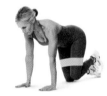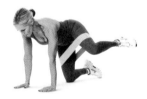

GLUTE BRIDGES

On your back with relaxed shoulders and neck, feet toward your bottom, tilt the pelvis toward you and drive up through the heels. Come down and repeat.

x 30 secs

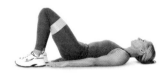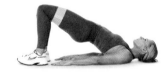

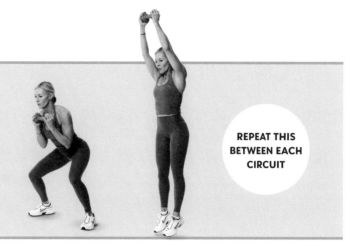

SQUAT JUMP AND PRESS

Start with a squat and when you get to the bottom of the squat, jump, bringing your legs together and press weight overhead. For a low-impact variation, take out the jump.

x 10 reps

REPEAT THIS BETWEEN EACH CIRCUIT

CIRCUIT 2

GOBLET SQUATS

Sumo squat with the feet wider, toes out, and weight close to the chest. Hips back with your weight through the heels, drive back up.

x 12 reps

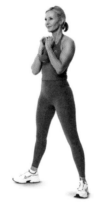
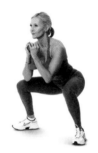

REVERSE LUNGES
(alternate legs)

With shoulders back and core engaged, step back to 90 degrees with one leg and power through the supporting heel to stand. Switch sides.

x 10 reps each side

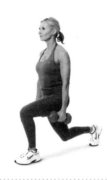
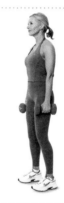

DEAD LIFTS

With a soft bend to the knee, hinge from the waist, sending the hips back straight and keeping the back straight. As soon as chest is parallel with the floor, drive up to stand. Try not to round through the spine or dip the head.

x 15 reps

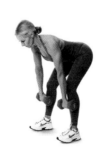
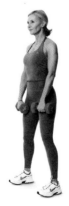

CIRCUIT 3

DONKEY KICKS

Start in a tabletop position, shoulders over wrists, abs tight. With foot flexed and knee bent, drive the foot to push away the ceiling. Don't twist the hips or go too high with the leg.

x 12 reps each side

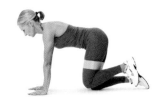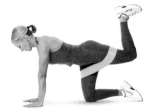

SPLIT SQUATS

Feet hip-width apart, shoulders back, core engaged, bend your knees so that they are 90 degrees to the ground (or wherever feels comfortable), chest lifted, front knee behind the toe. Come back to stand and repeat.

x 10 reps each side

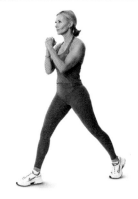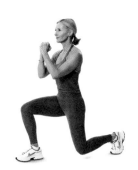

WALL SQUATS

With knees at 90 degrees and back against the wall, try not to let hands rest on the legs.

Hold x 30 secs

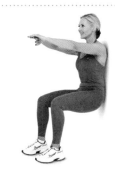

CIRCUIT 4

LATERAL LUNGES

Hips go back, chest lowers parallel to the thigh, other leg stays straight. Drive through the heel to push back to standing.

x 10 reps each side

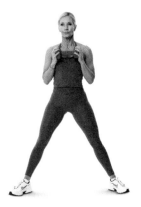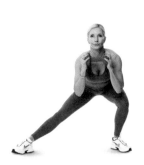

DUMBBELL SWINGS

All from the hips, knees are soft
(but not a squat), take the weight
between the legs and drive up to
shoulder height using the hips
to thrust forward.

x 15 reps

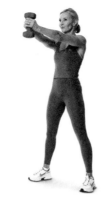
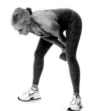

CIRCUIT 5
CORE

CRUNCHES

Bring your head and shoulders off
the mat, back down, supporting
the head without pulling on the
neck. Keep a space between the
chin and chest.

x 10 reps

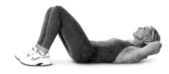
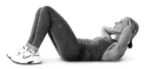

LOW PLANK DIPS

Keeping core strong and in a
straight line, slowly lower hips
from one side to the other.

x 10 reps

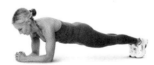
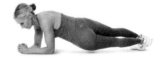

REVERSE CURLS

Keeping your head down, this is a
small movement, taking the hips
off the mat. Try to relax your neck
and shoulders.

x 10 reps

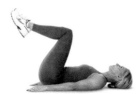
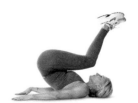

WEEK 04
FRIDAY

Rest x 15 secs between exercises and rest x 30 secs in between each circuit.

CIRCUIT 1
HIIT 3-MINUTE CARDIO
No repeats

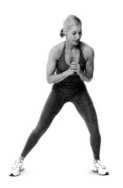
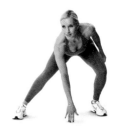

SHUTTLE RUNS
Take three strides across the mat, tapping down low at either end and bending knees while keeping the back straight.

x 30 secs

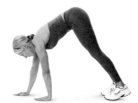
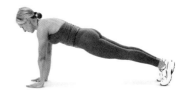

WALKOUTS
Keeping your legs straight, walk out your hands into a plank and then back to the starting position.

x 30 secs

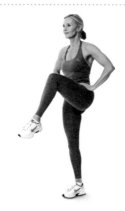

HIGH KNEES OR MARCHES
Standing tall, bring one knee up at a time, shoulders back.

x 30 secs

BURPEES

Start by standing with the arms by your side, feet shoulder-width apart. Bend the knees, squatting down to place the hands on the floor in front of the feet. Jump the legs back to a plank position with a straight line from the shoulders to the heels. Next, jump the legs back in and jump to return to standing. For a low-impact version step the legs in and out instead of jumping.

x 30 secs

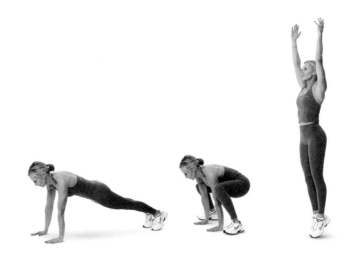

MOUNTAIN CLIMBERS

From a plank position, keep your hips down, back straight, core tight, shoulders over wrists, bring one knee into the chest and alternate. Do these at the right pace for you.

x 30 secs

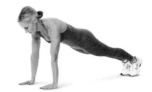
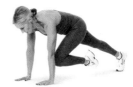

SQUATS OR SQUAT JUMPS

With all your weight in your heels, hips back, straight back, squat as if sitting into a chair, chest lifted, shoulders back. For high impact add a jump.

x 30 secs

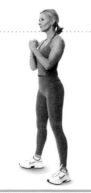
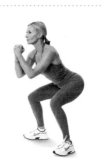

CIRCUIT 2
UPPER BODY

Repeat x 2 sets

REVERSE FLIES

Hinge from the hips, back straight and core tight. Slowly open the arms to shoulder height and, without swinging, slowly lower, palms facing in.

x 30 secs

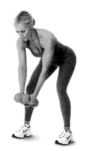
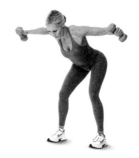

RENEGADE ROWS

In a plank position, avoid movement through the hips, drive the weight back close to your side (with elbows in) toward the back pocket of your leggings. Bottom down and straight back. You can start on your knees and progress to a plank.

x 30 secs

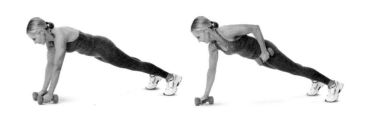

PUSH-UPS

With your hands wide on the mat, go down in one movement (without dipping the head), back straight and elbows back. Try to keep core engaged and come up in one movement. Start against the wall or a bench and progress to knees and on to toes.

x 30 secs

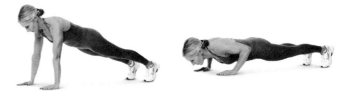

SHOULDER PRESSES

Knees soft, abs tight, keep elbows in line of vision. Slowly press the arms up and when lowered try to keep your elbows to 90 degrees.

x 30 secs

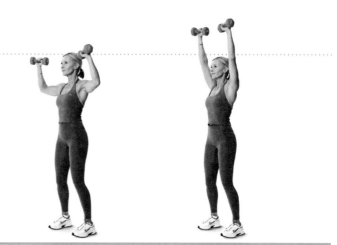

CIRCUIT 3
UPPER BODY CARDIO

Repeat x 3 sets

JABS

With core tight and knees soft, extend the arms, trying to keep the arms/weights at shoulder level.

x 20 secs

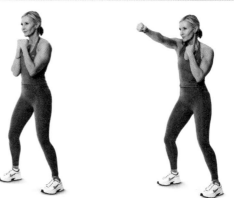

BURPEE INTO SHOULDER PRESS

Start by standing with the arms by your side, feet shoulder-width apart. Bend the knees, squatting down to place the hands on the floor in front of the feet. Jump the legs back to a plank position with a straight line from the shoulders to the heels. Next, jump the legs back in and as you stand you can either jump (body weight) or take your weights up into a shoulder press.

With your knees soft, abs tight, keep elbows in line of vision. Slowly press the arms up and when lowered, try to keep your elbows to 90 degrees.

x 20 secs

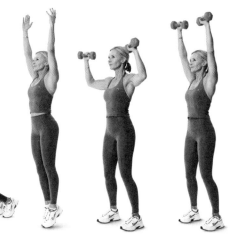

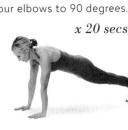

BEAR CRAWLS

Start in a plank position and walk in with the feet so that the knees stay under the hips. Keep back straight and bottom down. Shoulders stay over the wrists. Then walk back out to plank and repeat.

x 20 secs

CIRCUIT 4
LEGS

Repeat x 2 sets

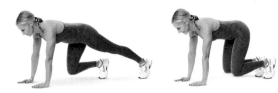

SNATCHES

Holding one weight in the center of the body, you squat down and then drive up with the weight—the other hand out to the side. Make it one movement and keep back straight. Switch sides.

x 30 secs each side

REVERSE LUNGES

(alternate legs)

With shoulders back and core engaged, step back to 90 degrees with one leg and power through the supporting heel to stand. Switch sides.

x 30 secs

DEADLIFTS

With a soft bend to the knee, hinge from the waist, sending the hips back and keeping the back straight. As soon as chest is parallel with the floor, drive up to stand. Try not to round through the spine or dip the head.

x 30 secs

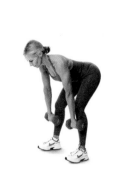
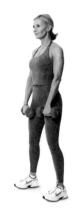

DONKEY KICKS

Start in a tabletop position, shoulders over wrists, abs tight. With foot flexed and knee bent, drive the foot to push away the ceiling. Don't twist the hips or go too high with the leg.

x 30 secs each side

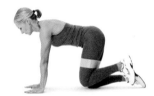
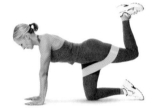

CIRCUIT 5
LOWER BODY CARDIO

Repeat x 3 sets

SQUAT JUMP AND PRESS

Start with a squat and when you get to the bottom of the squat, jump, bringing your legs together and press weight overhead (weight optional). For a low-impact variation, take out the jump.

x 20 secs

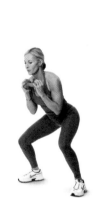
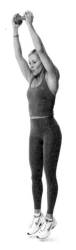

WALKOUTS

Keeping your legs straight, walk out your hands into a plank and then back to the starting position.

x 20 secs

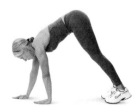
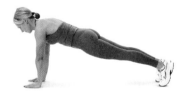

CROSS CLIMBERS

With shoulders over wrists and core engaged, bring each knee under the body toward the opposite elbow. Minimize movement through the hips and keep the back straight.

x 20 secs

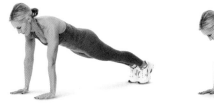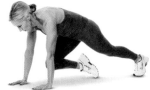

CIRCUIT 6
CORE

Repeat x 3 sets

BENT KNEE JACKKNIVES

Keeping back down, crunch into a ball and slowly extend arms and legs (only to where it feels comfortable).

x 20 secs

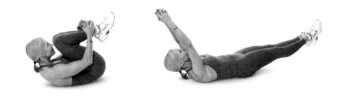

SIDE PLANK

(hold both sides)

With elbow directly under the shoulder, hold the position with core engaged and hips stacked (can be done on knees).

x 20 secs each side

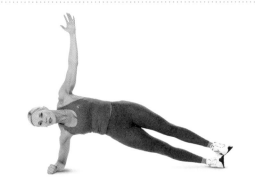

TOE TAPS

With your head off or down on the mat, bring your knees just above your hips and slowly lower each toe in turn to the mat. Ensure you keep your back down.

x 20 secs

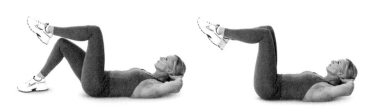

WEEK 05
MONDAY

30 MINS
FULL BODY
BANDS & WEIGHTS

Perform each exercise x 40 secs with x 15 secs rest betweeen each one—no repeats!

GOBLET SQUATS

Sumo squat with the feet wider, toes out, and weight close to the chest. Hips back with your weight through the heels, drive back up.

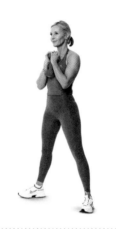
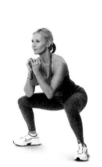

RENEGADE ROWS

In a plank position, avoid movement through the hips, drive the weight back close to your side (with elbows in) toward the back pocket of your leggings. Bottom down and straight back. You can start on your knees and progress to a plank.

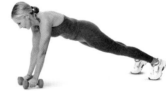
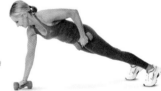

BENT-OVER ROWS

Hinge from the hips, with arms extended for full range of motion. Keep back straight and the head in line with the spine. Slowly bring arms back toward the pocket of your leggings. Core tight. Do not round spine.

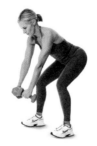
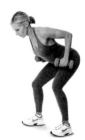

ALTERNATE FRONT RAISES

Slowly raise each arm alternately, without swinging or leaning back. Keep knees soft and shoulders back, chest lifted.

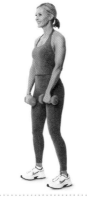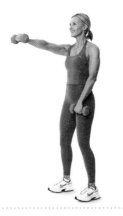

SPLIT SQUATS

(each side)

Feet hip-width apart, shoulders back, core engaged, bend your knees so that they are 90 degrees to the ground (or wherever feels comfortable), chest lifted, front knee behind the toe. Come back to stand and repeat.

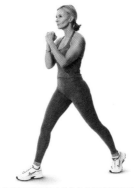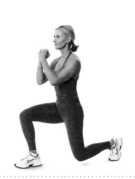

DEADLIFT INTO REVERSE LUNGE

(alternate legs)

With a soft bend to the knee, hinge from the waist, sending the hips back, keeping the back straight. As soon as chest is parallel with the floor, drive up to stand. Try not to round through the spine or dip the head. With shoulders back and core engaged, step back to 90 degrees with the leg and power through the supporting heel to stand. Switch sides.

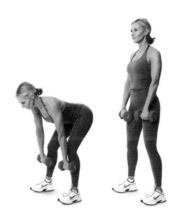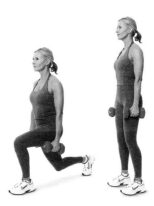

ZOTTMAN CURLS

Bicep curl on the way up, turn the wrists at the top, and slowly lower, with elbows locked into your sides.

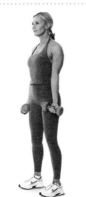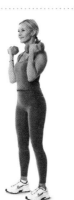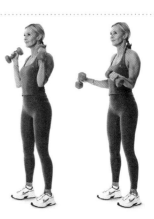

CHEST PRESSES

Keeping your elbows in your peripheral vision, imagine the letter "A" and press arms above chest (not the head), breathing out on the exertion.

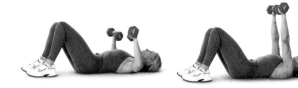

OPEN CHEST FLIES

Lie on your back with your head on the ground. Keep a slight bend to the elbows—open the arms, without resting on the mat, as you take them wide and then drive back to the starting position over the chest.

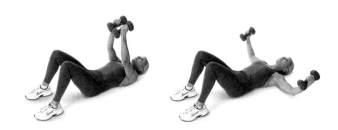

PUSH-UPS

With your hands wide on the mat, go down in one movement (without dipping the head), back straight and elbows back. Try to keep core engaged and come up in one movement. Start against the wall or a bench and progress to knees and on to toe.

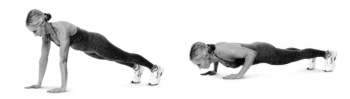

SLOW MOUNTAIN CLIMBERS

From a plank position, keep your hips down, back straight, core tight, shoulders over wrists, bring one knee into the chest and alternate. Do these at the right pace for you.

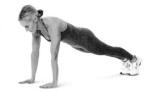
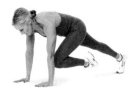

CURTSY LUNGES

(each side)

Take one leg diagonally behind without twisting the front knee, keep upright with the body, and bend down as far with the back knee as is comfortable. Come back to stand and repeat.

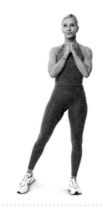
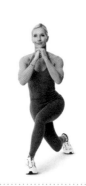

SINGLE ARNOLD SHOULDER PRESS

(each side)

With elbows out in front of you at shoulder height, slowly move one arm out to the side, extend into a a shoulder press, lower again, and as you lower the arm, turn the palm back to face you. Repeat.

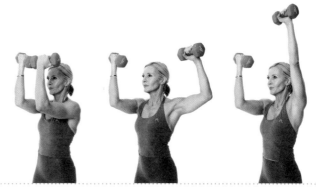

SQUAT AND PRESS

Lower into the squat position and as you come back to standing raise the arms into a shoulder press.

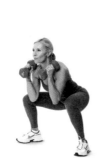
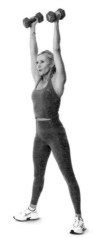

OVERHEAD TRICEP EXTENSIONS

Standing or kneeling with arms above your head, keep elbows close to ears as you bend the arms back. Slowly return to starting position. Don't lean back.

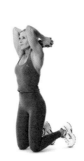
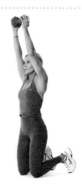

WIDE CURLS

With elbows tucked in, shoulders back, core engaged, and arms bent outward, use your biceps as you bend the arms at the elbow and lift toward the shoulders. Slowly on the way up and on the way down.

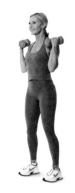
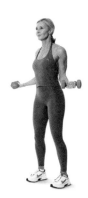

DUMBBELL SWINGS

All from the hips, knees are soft (but not a squat), take the weight between the legs and drive up to shoulder height using the hips to thrust forward.

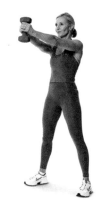
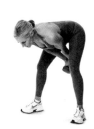

BICYCLE CRUNCHES

Without pulling on your head, bring opposite elbow to opposite knee, keeping your back down. Slowly extend the leg and switch sides. Go slowly to work the obliques without momentum.

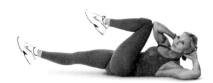

DEAD BUGS

On your back, head down or off the mat, extend the opposite arm and opposite leg slowly before returning to start position. Switch sides. Keep the back on the floor and core engaged throughout. You can also do this with light weights.

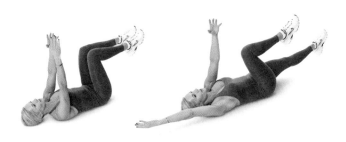

GLUTE BRIDGES

On your back with relaxed
shoulders and neck, feet toward
your bottom, tilt the pelvis
toward you and drive up
through the heels. Come
down and repeat.

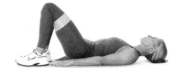 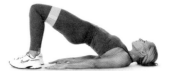

JABS

With core tight and knees
soft, extend the arms, trying to
keep the arms/weights at
shoulder level.

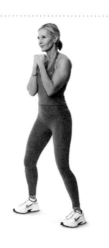 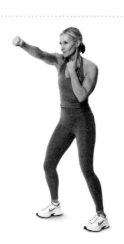

BEAR CRAWLS

Start in a plank position and walk in
with the feet so that the knees stay
under the hips. Keep back straight
and bottom down. Shoulders stay
over the wrists. Then walk back
out to plank and repeat.

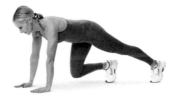 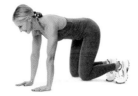

COMMANDOS

Starting in high plank, lower down
into low plank, try to keep hips still,
then push back to a high plank
position and change direction.

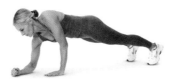 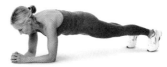

WEEK 05
TUESDAY

Repeat x 2 sets. Rest x 20 secs between exercises. Perform tricep dips in between each circuit x 30 secs.

SUPERSET 1

TRICEP PUSH-UPS

Unlike a chest push up, hands are narrower on the mat; go down in one movement (without dipping the head), back straight and elbows tucked in. Try to keep core engaged and come up in one movement. Start against the wall or a bench and progress to knees and on to toes.

x 40 secs

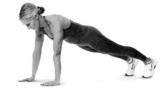

OVERHEAD TRICEP EXTENSIONS

Standing or kneeling with arms above your head, bend your arms back keeping elbows close to ears. Slowly return to starting position. Don't lean back.

x 40 secs

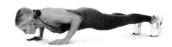

TRICEP DIPS

Keeping your back close to the surface of the chair, lower your body until your elbows are at 90 degrees, hands pointing, forward then come back up.

x 30 secs

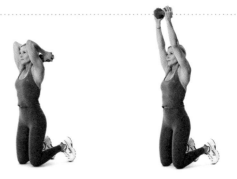
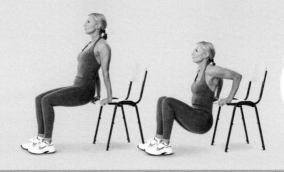

REPEAT THIS BETWEEN EACH CIRCUIT

SUPERSET 2

BICEP CURLS

Trying not to swing the arms, with your elbows locked into your side, slowly lift the weights and lower to the bottom and repeat.

x 40 secs

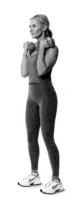
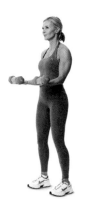

WIDE CURLS

With elbows tucked in, shoulders back, core engaged, and arms bent outward, use your biceps as you bend the arms at the elbow and lift toward the shoulders. Slowly on the way up and on the way down.

x 40 secs

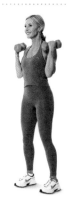
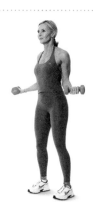

SUPERSET 3

TRICEP KICKBACKS

In a tabletop position, slowly extend the arm to the line of your body without swinging. Avoid twisting the hips and keep the back straight, shoulders over wrists.

x 30 secs each side

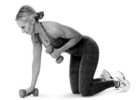
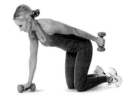

SKULL CRUSHERS

Lying down—using one weight or two—keep elbows tucked in as you take the weight behind the head. Bring back to starting position and repeat. Only the lower part of the arm moves.

x 40 secs

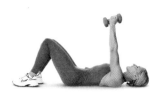
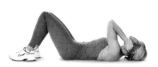

SUPERSET 4

ZOTTMAN CURLS

Bicep curl on the way up, turn the
wrists at the top, and slowly lower,
with elbows locked into your sides.

x 40 secs

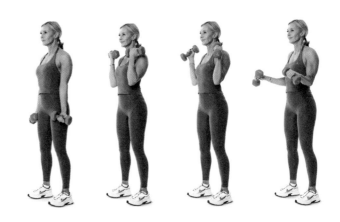

BICEP CURLS

Trying not to swing the arms, with
your elbows locked into your side,
slowly lift the weights and lower
to the bottom and repeat.

x 30 secs

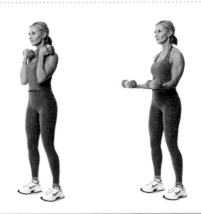

TO FINISH

SINGLE ARNOLD
SHOULDER PRESS

(each side)

With elbows out in front of you at
shoulder height, slowly move one
arm out to the side, extend into a
a shoulder press, lower again and
as you lower the arm, turn the
palm back to face you. Repeat.

x 30 secs each side

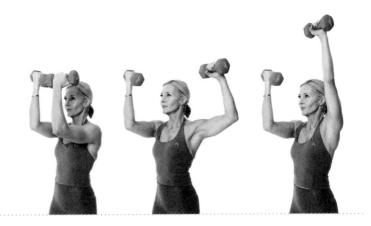

PLANK HOLD *(high or low)*

Shoulders over the wrists in either
high or low plank position, bottom
down, core tight. Glutes engaged.
Back straight.

Hold x 40 secs

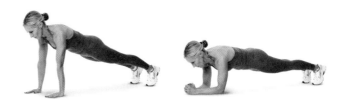

WEEK 05
WEDNESDAY

30 MINS
LOWER BODY
BANDS & WEIGHTS

No repeats! Go heavy if you can. Unless stated, every exercise is x 40 secs with x 20 secs rest.

CIRCUIT 1
LEGS

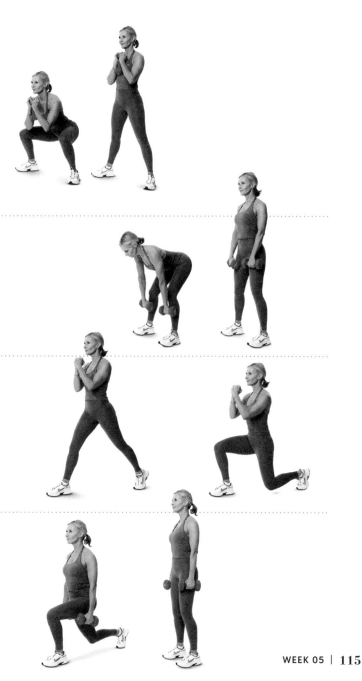

GOBLET SQUATS

Sumo squat with the feet wider, toes out, and weight close to the chest. Hips back with your weight through the heels, drive back up.

DEADLIFTS

With a soft bend to the knee, hinge from the hips, sending them back and keeping the back straight. As soon as the chest is parallel with the floor, drive up to stand. Try not to round through the spine or dip the head.

SPLIT SQUATS (each side)

Feet hip-width apart, shoulders back, core engaged, bend your knees so that they are 90 degrees to the ground (or wherever feels comfortable), chest lifted, front knee behind the toe. Come back to stand and repeat.

REVERSE LUNGES (alternate legs)

With shoulders back and core engaged, step back to 90 degrees with one leg and power through the supporting heel to stand. Switch sides.

GLUTE BRIDGES

On your back with relaxed shoulders and neck, feet toward your bottom, tilt the pelvis toward you and drive up through the heels. Come down and repeat.

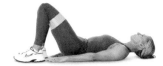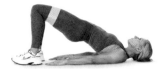

STANDING LEG RAISES

(each side)

Keep the knee of the supporting leg slightly bent, stand upright and with foot flexed slowly raise the leg straight up to the side (not too high) and lower back to standing.

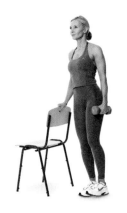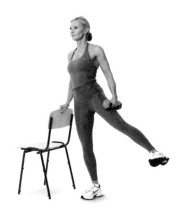

GOBLET SQUATS
WITH 3 PULSES

Sumo squat with the feet wider, toes out, and weight close to the chest. Hips back with your weight through the heels, stay low for 3 pulses before driving back up.

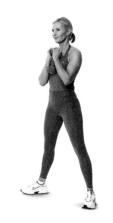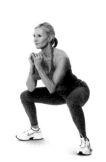

CURTSY LUNGES

Take one leg diagonally behind without twisting the front knee, keep upright with the body, and bend down as far with the back knee as is comfortable. Come back to stand and repeat.

x 20 secs each side.

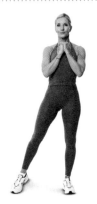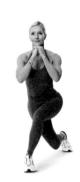

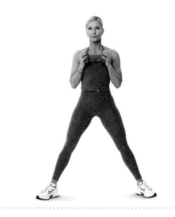
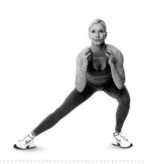

LATERAL LUNGES

(both sides)

Hips go back, chest lowers parallel to the thigh, other leg stays straight. Drive through the heel to push back to standing. Switch sides.

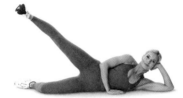
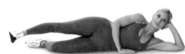

SIDE-LYING LEG RAISES

(both sides)

In a straight line with hips stacked and lower leg bent, slowly raise the top leg with foot flexed and slowly lower. Keep the core engaged.

1 DEADLIFT INTO 2 REVERSE LUNGES

(alternate legs)

With a soft bend to the knee, hinge from the waist, sending the hips back, keeping the back straight. As soon as the chest is parallel with the floor, drive up to stand. Try not to round through the spine or dip the head. Then, with shoulders back and core engaged, step back to 90 degrees with one leg and power through the supporting heel to stand. Switch sides.

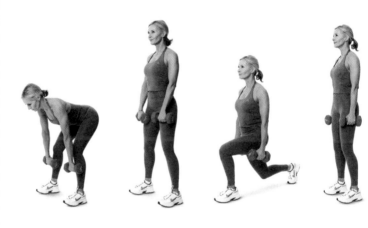

BODY-WEIGHT SQUATS (20 secs) & SQUAT JUMPS (20 secs)

With all your weight in your heels, hips back, straight back, squat as if sitting into a chair, chest lifted, shoulders back. For body-weight squats, return to standing. For squat jump, jump to return to start position.

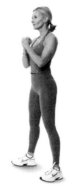
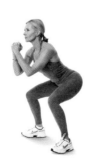

CIRCUIT 2
CORE

CRUNCHES

Bring your head and shoulders off the mat, back down, supporting the head without pulling on the neck. Keep a space between the chin and chest.

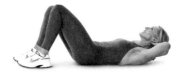 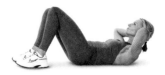

SIDE PLANK HOLD

With elbow directly under the shoulder, hold the position with core engaged and hips stacked (can be done on knees).

Hold x 30 secs each side

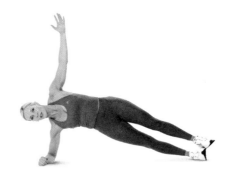

LEG EXTENSIONS

With your back down, only lower legs to where it feels comfortable and without your back coming off the floor.

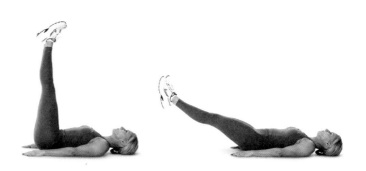

PLANK SHOULDER TAPS

Start with shoulders over wrists, back straight, abs engaged, and head in line with spine. Slowly tap your hand to each shoulder in turn, trying to avoid movement through the hips. Squeeze the glutes.

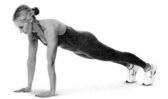 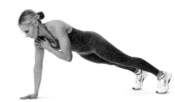

BENT KNEE JACKKNIVES

Keeping back down, crunch into a ball and slowly extend arms and legs (only to where it feels comfortable).

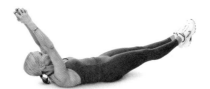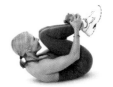

LOW PLANK DIPS

Keeping core strong and in a straight line, slowly lower hips from one side to the other.

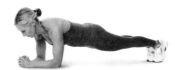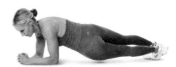

BICYCLE CRUNCHES

Without pulling on your head, bring opposite elbow to knee, keeping your back down. Slowly extend the leg and switch sides. Go slowly to work the obliques without momentum.

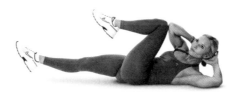

TOE TAPS

With your head off or down on the mat, bring your knees just above your hips and slowly lower each toe in turn to the mat. Ensure you keep your back down.

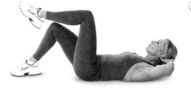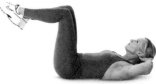

WEEK 05
FRIDAY

30 MINS
STRENGTH HIIT
WEIGHTS

All exercises performed for x 30 secs with x 10 secs rest in between each. Perform shuttle runs x 40 secs between each circuit.

CIRCUIT 1
3 x sets

DUMBBELL SWINGS

All from the hips, knees are soft (but not a squat), take the weight between the legs and drive up to shoulder height using the hips to thrust forward.

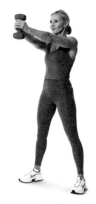 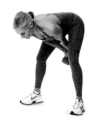

REVERSE LUNGES

(alternate legs)

With shoulders back and core engaged, step back to 90 degrees with one leg and power through the supporting heel to stand. Switch sides.

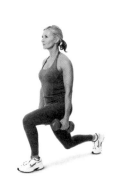 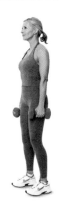

MOUNTAIN CLIMBERS

From a plank position, keep your hips down, back straight, core tight, shoulders over wrists, bring one knee into the chest and alternate. Do these at the right pace for you.

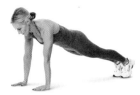 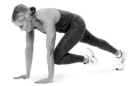

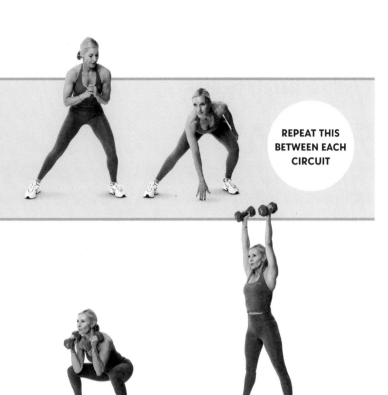

SHUTTLE RUNS

Take three strides across the mat, tapping down low at either end and bending knees while keeping the back straight.

x 40 secs

REPEAT THIS BETWEEN EACH CIRCUIT

CIRCUIT 2

3 x sets

SQUAT AND PRESS

Lower into the squat position and as you come back to standing raise the arms into a shoulder press.

RENEGADE ROWS

In a plank position, avoid movement through the hips, drive the weight back close to your side (with elbows in) toward the back pocket of your leggings. Bottom down and straight back. You can start on your knees and progress to a plank.

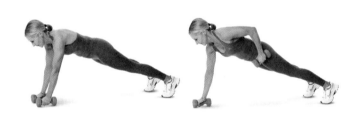

BURPEES

Start by standing with the arms by your side, feet shoulder-width apart. Bend the knees, squatting down to place the hands on the floor in front of the feet. Jump the legs back to a plank position with a straight line from the shoulders to the heels. Next, jump the legs back in and jump to return to standing. For a low-impact version, step the legs in and out instead of jumping.

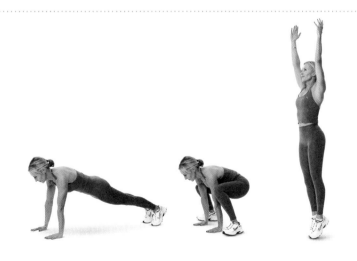

CIRCUIT 3

2 x sets

SNATCHES

Holding one weight in the center of the body, you squat down and then drive up with the weight—the other hand out to the side. Make it one movement and keep back straight. Switch sides.

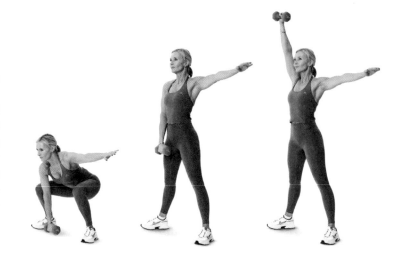

DEADLIFTS

With a soft bend to the knee, hinge from the hips, sending them back and keeping the back straight. As soon as the chest is parallel with the floor, drive up to stand. Try not to round through the spine or dip the head.

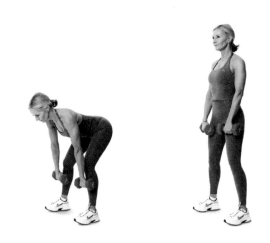

JABS

With core tight and knees soft, extend the arms, trying to keep the arms/weights at shoulder level.

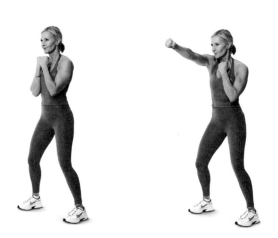

CIRCUIT 4
AMRAP

Timer set to 4 mins

CROSS CLIMBERS

With shoulders over wrists and core engaged, bring each knee under the body toward the opposite elbow. Minimize movement through the hips and keep the back straight.

x 20 reps

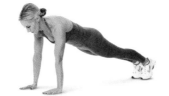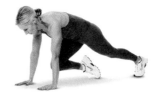

BENT KNEE JACKKINVES

Keeping back down, crunch into a ball and slowly extend arms and legs (only to where it feels comfortable).

x 10 reps

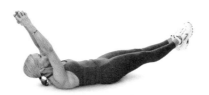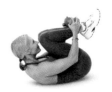

REVERSE CURLS

Keeping your head down, this is a small movement, taking the hips off the mat. Try to relax your neck and shoulders.

x 10 reps

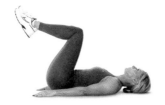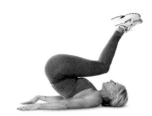

RUSSIAN TWISTS

Feet can stay down or come off the mat. Slowly turn from side to side without moving the knees. Keep abs tight throughout. Perform with or without weights.

x 10 reps

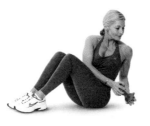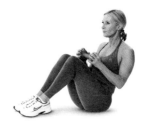

WEEK 06
MONDAY

Perform each exercise for x 45 secs with x 15 secs rest between exercises (circuits 1 and 3 only). Repeat each circuit x 2 sets.

CIRCUIT 1

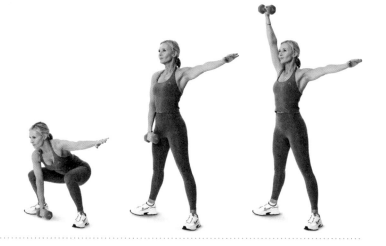

SNATCHES

Holding one weight in the center of the body, you squat down and then drive up with the weight—the other hand out to the side. Make it one movement and keep back straight. Switch sides.

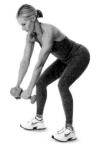
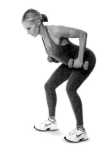

BENT-OVER ROWS

Hinge from the hips, with arms extended for full range of motion. Keep back straight and the head in line with the spine. Slowly bring arms back toward the pocket of your leggings. Core tight. Do not round spine.

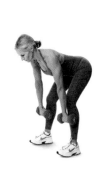
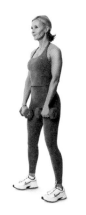
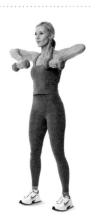

DEADLIFT INTO UPRIGHT ROW

With a soft bend to the knee, hinge from the hips, sending them back and keeping the back straight. As soon as the chest is parallel with the floor, drive up to stand. Try not to round through the spine or dip the head. Bring the arms farther up into an upright row for the shoulders.

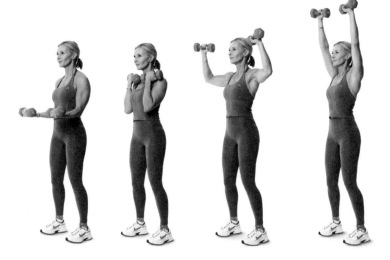

BICEP CURL INTO SHOULDER PRESS

Trying not to swing the arms, with your elbows locked into your side, slowly lift the weights into a bicep curl and then take the weights overhead into a shoulder press.

SKULL CRUSHERS

Lying down—using one weight or two—keep elbows tucked in as you take the weight behind the head. Bring back to starting position and repeat. Only the lower part of the arm moves.

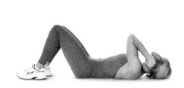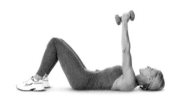

PLANK WITH SHOULDER TAPS OR COMMANDOS

Start with shoulders over wrists, back straight, abs engaged, and head in line with spine. Slowly tap your hand to each shoulder in turn, trying to avoid movement through the hips.

Alternatively, for commandos, lower down into low plank, try to keep hips still, then push back to a high plank position.

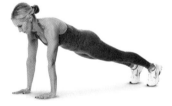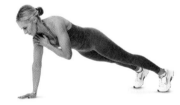

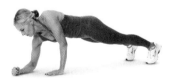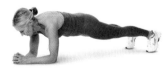

CIRCUIT 2
4 MINUTES, EMOM

Perform the first exercise for
x 10 reps, then the second exercise
for the rest of the minute.

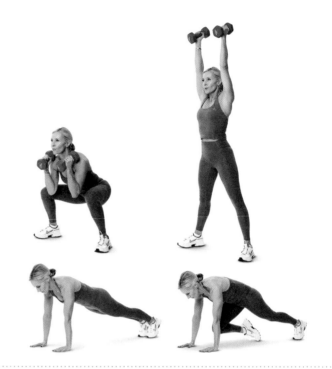

SQUAT AND PRESS
INTO CROSS CLIMBERS

Lower into the squat position and as you come back to standing raise the arms into a shoulder press.

With shoulders over wrists and core engaged, bring each knee under the body toward the opposite elbow. Minimize movement through the hips and keep the back straight.

SLOW RENEGADE ROWS
INTO DUMBBELL SWINGS

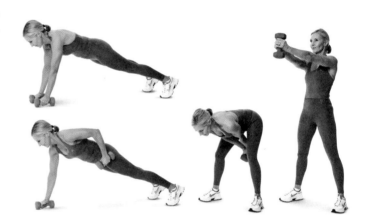

In a plank position, avoid movement through the hips, drive the weight back close to your side (with elbows in) toward the back pocket of your leggings. Bottom down and straight back. You can start on your knees and progress to a plank.

With soft knees and all movement from the hips, take the weight between the legs and drive up to shoulder height. Using the hips to thrust forward squeeze the glutes.

CHEST PRESSES
INTO RUSSIAN TWISTS

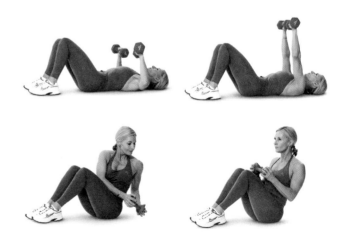

Keeping your elbows in your peripheral vision, imagine the letter "A" and press arms above chest (not the head), breathing out on the exertion.

Feet can stay down or come off the mat. Slowly turn from side to side without moving the knees. Keep abs tight throughout and look right around to each side. Perform with or without weights.

SPLIT SQUATS (x 10 each side)
INTO SQUAT JUMPS

Feet hip-width apart, shoulders back, core engaged, bend your knees so that they are 90 degrees to the ground (or wherever it feels comfortable), chest lifted, front knee behind the toe. Return to standing position and repeat on other side, before moving onto a squat jump (below).

With all your weight in your heels, hips back, straight back, squat as if sitting into a chair, chest lifted, shoulders back. For high impact add a jump.

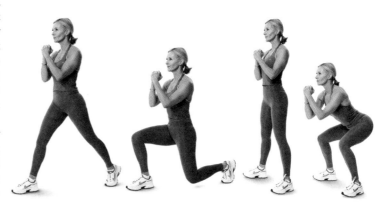

CIRCUIT 3
CORE

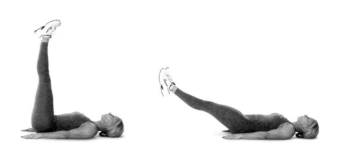

LEG EXTENSIONS

With your back down, only lower legs to where it feels comfortable and without your back coming off the floor.

LOW PLANK DIPS

Keep core strong and in a straight line, slowly lower hips from one side to the other.

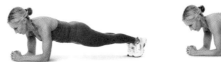
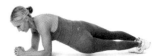

CRUNCHES

Bring your head and shoulders off the mat, back down, supporting the head without pulling on the neck. Keep a space between the chin and chest.

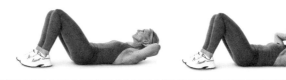

BEAR CRAWLS

Start in a plank position and walk in with the feet so that the knees stay under the hips. Keep back straight and bottom down. Shoulders stay over the wrists. Then walk back out to plank and repeat.

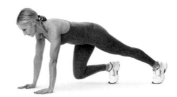
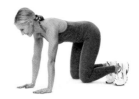

WEEK 06
TUESDAY

Rest x 20 secs between exercises. Perform push-ups in between each circuit (knees or toes).

CIRCUIT 1
CHEST

Repeat x 3 sets

CHEST PRESSES

Keeping your elbows in your peripheral vision, imagine the letter "A" and press arms above chest (not the head), breathing out on the exertion.

x 40 secs

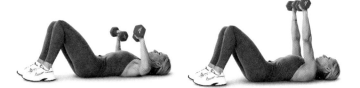

OPEN CHEST FLIES

Lie on your back with your head on the ground. Keep a slight bend to the elbows—open the arms, without resting on the mat, as you take them wide and then drive back to the starting position over the chest.

x 20 secs

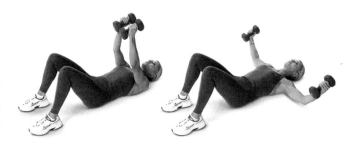

PUSH-UPS

With your hands wide on the mat, go down in one movement (without dipping the head), back straight and elbows back. Try to keep core engaged and come up in one movement.

x 10 reps

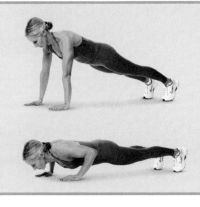

REPEAT THIS BETWEEN EACH CIRCUIT

CIRCUIT 2
BACK

Repeat x 2 sets

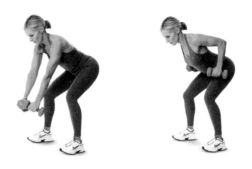

BENT-OVER ROWS

Hinge from the hips, with arms extended for full range of motion. Keep back straight and the head in line with the spine. Slowly bring arms back toward the pocket of your leggings. Core tight. Do not round spine.

x 40 secs

REVERSE FLIES

Hinge from the hips, back straight and core tight. Slowly open the arms to shoulder height and, without swinging, slowly lower, palms facing in.

x 20 secs

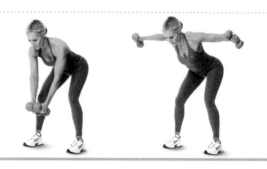

CIRCUIT 3
SHOULDERS

Repeat x 2 sets

SINGLE ARNOLD SHOULDER PRESSES *(each side)*

Seated or standing, with elbows out in front of you at shoulder height, slowly move one arm out to the side, extend into a shoulder press, lower again, and as you lower the arm, turn the palm back to face you. Repeat.

x 40 secs

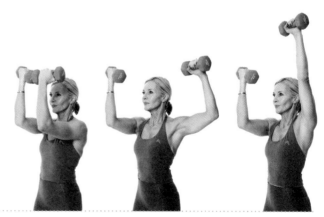

AIRPLANES

Using light or no weights, try to keep the arms at shoulder height and draw little circles in one direction and then the other.

x 20 secs

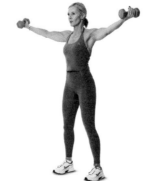

CIRCUIT 4
BICEPS

Repeat x 2 sets

BICEP CURLS

Trying not to swing the arms, with your elbows locked into your side, slowly lift the weights and lower to the bottom and repeat.

x 40 secs

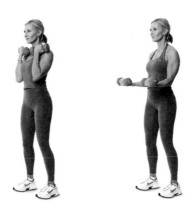

ZOTTMAN CURLS

Bicep curl on the way up, turn the wrists at the top and slowly lower, with elbows locked into your sides.

x 20 secs

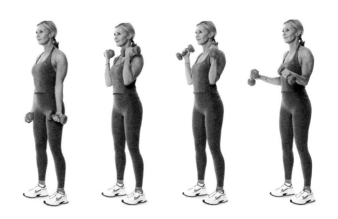

CIRCUIT 5
TRICEPS

Repeat x 2 sets

OVERHEAD TRICEP EXTENSIONS

Standing or kneeling with arms above your head, bend your arm back keeping elbows close to ears. Slowly return to starting position. Don't lean back.

x 40 secs

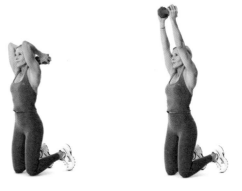

TRICEP DIPS

Keeping your back close to the surface of the chair, lower your body until your elbows are at 90 degrees, hands pointing forward, then come back up.

x 20 secs

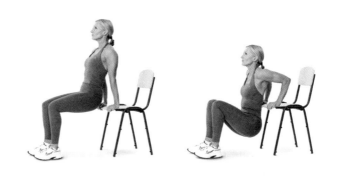

TO FINISH
CORE / TABATA

*10 x secs rest
between each exercise*

COMMANDOS

Starting in high plank, lower down into low plank, try to keep hips still, then push back to a high plank position and change direction.

x 20 secs

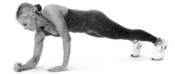 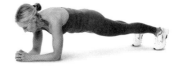

LEG EXTENSIONS

With your back down, only lower legs to where it feels comfortable and without your back coming off the floor.

x 20 secs

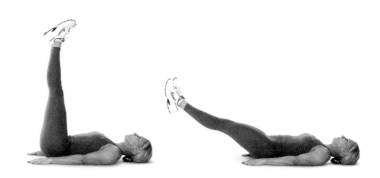

CRUNCHES

Bring your head and shoulders off the mat, back down, supporting the head without pulling on the neck. Keep a space between the chin and chest.

x 20 secs

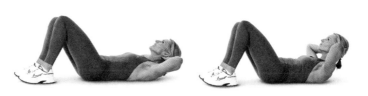

WEEK 06
WEDNESDAY

Rest x 15 secs between exercises.

CIRCUIT 1
Repeat x 2 sets

GOBLET SQUATS

Sumo squat with the feet wider, toes out, and weight close to the chest. Hips back with your weight through the heels, drive back up.

x 40 secs

SQUAT WITH 5 PULSES

With all your weight in your heels, hips back, straight back, squat as if sitting into a chair, chest lifted, shoulders back. Stay low for 5 pulses before returning to stand.

x 40 secs

CURTSY LUNGES

Take one leg diagonally behind without twisting the front knee, keep upright with the body, and bend down as far with the back knee as is comfortable. Come back to stand and repeat.

x 30 secs each side

LATERAL LUNGES

Hips go back, chest lowers parallel to the thigh, other leg stays straight. Drive through the heel to push back to standing. Switch sides.

x 40 secs each side

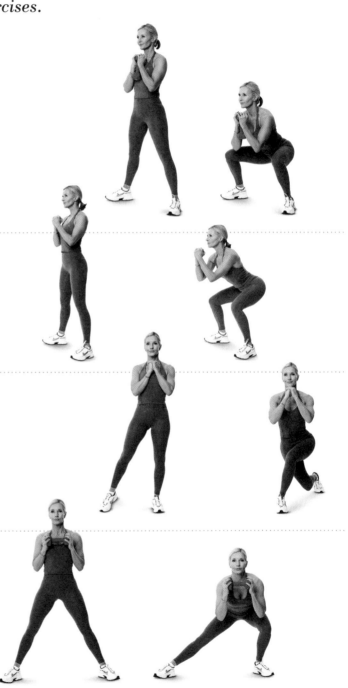

GLUTE BRIDGES

On your back with relaxed shoulders and neck, feet toward your bottom, tilt the pelvis toward you and drive up through the heels. Come down and repeat.

x 40 secs

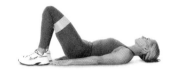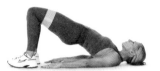

SPLIT SQUATS

Feet hip-width apart, shoulders back, core engaged, bend your knees so that they are 90 degrees to the ground (or wherever it feels comfortable), chest lifted, front knee behind the toe. Come back to stand and repeat.

x 30 secs each side

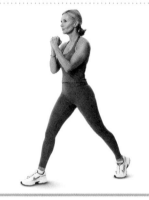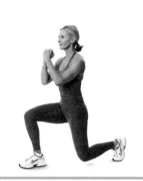

CIRCUIT 2

Repeat x 2 sets

FIRE HYDRANTS

In a tabletop position without twisting the hips, slowly raise one knee to the side and slowly lower.

x 30 secs each side

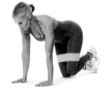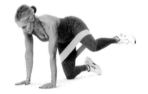

DONKEY KICKS

Start in a tabletop position, shoulders over wrists, abs tight. With foot flexed and knee bent, drive the foot to push away the ceiling. Don't twist the hips or go too high with the leg.

x 30 secs each side

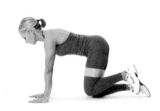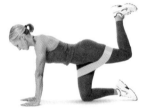

CLAMSHELLS

Lie on your side on the mat. Keep your feet together at the heel. Slowly raise the top knee, squeezing the glutes and slowly lower. Hips stay stacked and upper body lifted, abs engaged.

x 30 secs each side

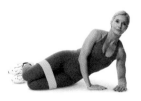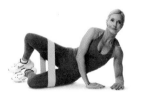

SIDE-LYING LEG RAISES

In a straight line with hips stacked and lower leg bent, slowly raise the top leg with foot flexed and slowly lower. Keep the core engaged.

x 30 secs each side

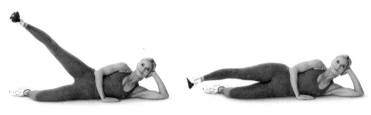

CIRCUIT 3

Repeat x 1 set

GLUTE KICKBACKS

From a tabletop position, with the core engaged, lift your leg behind you and squeeze glutes. (Don't take the leg too high.)

x 30 secs each side

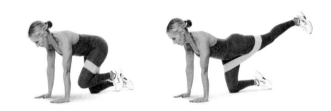

SQUAT PULSES

With all your weight in your heels, hips back, straight back, squat as if sitting into a chair, chest lifted, shoulders back. Stay low at the bottom and pulse for the duration of the exercise

x 40 secs

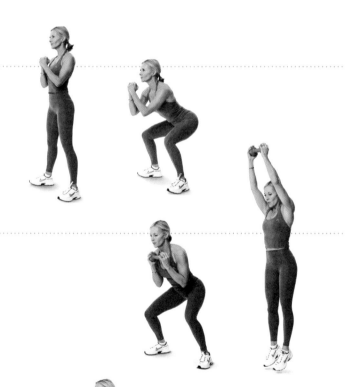

SQUAT JUMP AND PRESS

Start with a squat and when you get to the bottom of the squat, jump, bringing your legs together and press weight overhead (weight optional). For a low-impact variation, take out jump.

x 10 reps

WALL SQUATS

With knees at 90 degrees and back against the wall, try not to let hands rest on the legs.

Hold x 50 secs

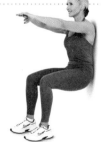

CIRCUIT 4
CORE

CRUNCHES

Bring your head and shoulders off the mat, back down, supporting the head without pulling on the neck. Keep a space between the chin and chest,

x 30 secs

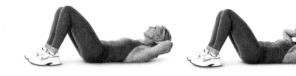

BICYCLE CRUNCHES

Without pulling on your head, bring opposite elbow to opposite knee, keeping your back down. Slowly extend the leg and switch sides. Go slowly to work the obliques without momentum.

x 30 secs

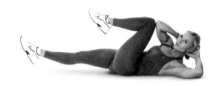

REVERSE CURLS

Keeping your head down, this is a small movement, taking the hips off the mat. Try to relax your neck and shoulders.

x 30 secs

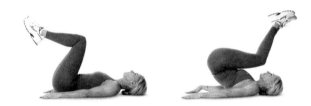

MOUNTAIN CLIMBERS

From a plank position, keep your hips down, back straight, core tight, shoulders over wrists, bring one knee into the chest and alternate. Do these at the right pace for you.

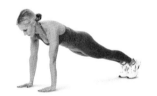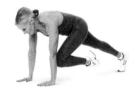

PLANK HOLD
(high or low)

Shoulders over the wrists in either high or low plank position, bottom down, core tight. Glutes engaged. Back straight.

Hold x 30 secs

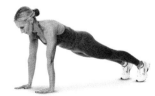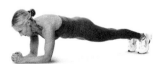

WEEK 06
FRIDAY

3 x sets of each circuit: x 40 secs for set 1, x 30 secs for set 2, x 20 secs for set 3. Rest x 15 secs between exercises.

CIRCUIT 1

SNATCHES

Holding one weight in the center of the body, you squat down and then drive up with the weight—the other hand out to the side. Make it one movement and keep back straight. Switch sides.

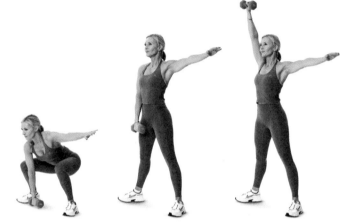

REVERSE LUNGE INTO BICEP CURL

With shoulders back and core engaged, step back to 90 degrees with one leg and power through the supporting heel to stand. As you come back to stand perform a bicep curl with your elbows locked in. Return to start and switch sides.

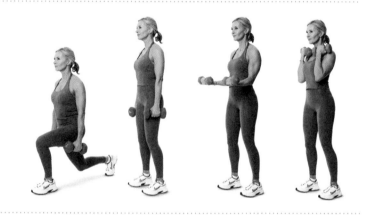

DUMBBELL SWINGS

All from the hips, knees are soft (but not a squat), take the weight between the legs and drive up to shoulder height using the hips to thrust forward.

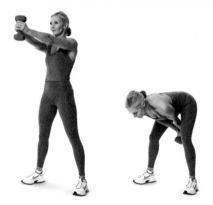

BURPEES

Start by standing with the arms by your side, feet shoulder-width apart. Bend the knees, squatting down to place the hands on the floor in front of the feet. Jump the legs back to a plank position with a straight line from the shoulders to the heels. Next, jump the legs back in and jump to return to standing. For a low-impact version step the legs in and out instead of jumping.

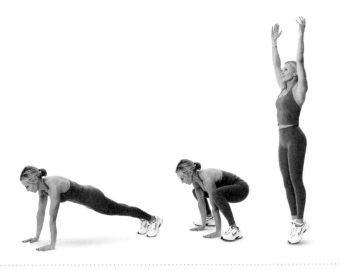

CIRCUIT 2

GOBLET SQUATS WITH 3 PULSES

Sumo squat with the feet wider, toes out, and weight close to the chest. Hips back with your weight through the heels, stay low for 3 pulses before driving back up.

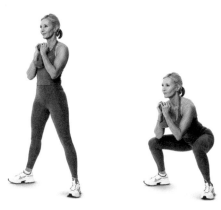

RENEGADE ROWS

In a plank position, avoid movement through the hips, drive the weight back close to your side (with elbows in) toward the back pocket of your leggings. Bottom down and straight back. You can start on your knees and progress to a plank.

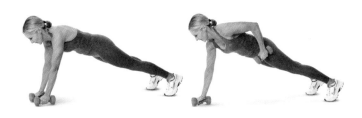

MOUNTAIN CLIMBERS

From a plank position, keep your hips down, back straight, core tight, shoulders over wrists, bring one knee into the chest and alternate. Do these at the right pace for you.

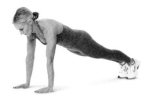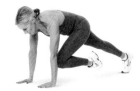

CIRCUIT 3

SQUAT AND PRESS

Lower into the squat position and as you come back to standing raise the arms into a shoulder press.

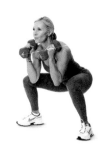
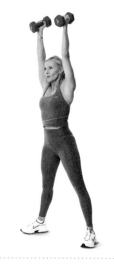

PUSH-UPS

With your hands wide on the mat, go down in one movement (without dipping the head), back straight and elbows back. Try to keep core engaged and come up in one movement. Start against the wall or a bench and progress to knees and on to toes.

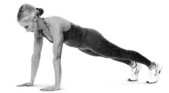
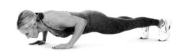

TO FINISH
CORE

20 x secs, back-to-back, no repeats

RUSSIAN TWISTS

Feet can stay down or come off the mat. Slowly turn from side to side without moving the knees. Keep abs tight throughout. Perform with or without weights.

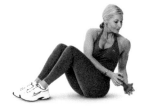
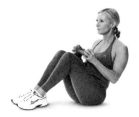

BENT KNEE JACKKNIVES

Keeping back down, crunch into a ball and slowly extend arms and legs (only to where it feels comfortable).

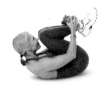
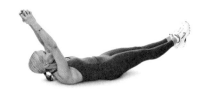

LOW PLANK DIPS

Keeping core strong and in a straight line, slowly lower hips from one side to the other.

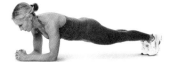 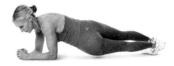

TOE TAPS

With your head off or down on the mat, bring your knees just above your hips and slowly lower each toe in turn to the mat. Ensure you keep your back down.

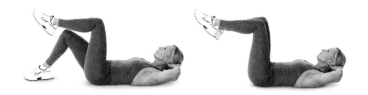

LEG EXTENSIONS

With your back down, only lower legs to where it feels comfortable and without your back coming off the floor.

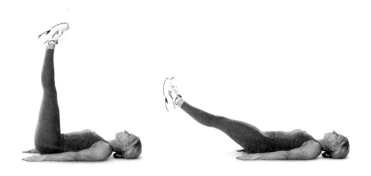

BEAR CRAWLS

Start in a plank position and walk in with the feet so that the knees stay under the hips. Keep back straight and bottom down. Shoulders stay over the wrists. Then walk back out to plank and repeat.

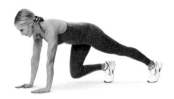 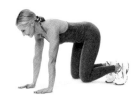

COMMANDOS

Starting in high plank, lower down into low plank, try to keep hips still, then push back to a high plank position and change direction.

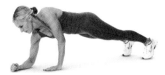 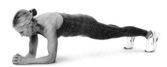

EXERCISE
MODIFICATIONS

Here are some common exercises and an alternative option for each one. Never be afraid to modify an exercise in a workout, as it's important to build strength at your own pace and with correct technique to avoid injury. These are also useful if you have an existing injury and need to replace one exercise with another.

DO YOU FIND IT HARD TO DO PUSH-UPS?

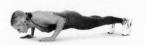 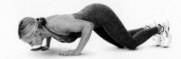

Start with push-ups on your knees or against the wall while you increase your upper body strength.

DO YOU SUFFER FROM WRIST PAIN WITH TRICEP DIPS?

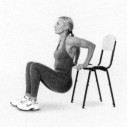 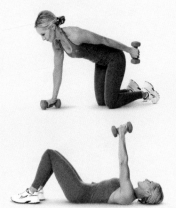

Replace with tricep kickbacks (see page 68) instead.

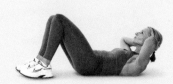

Or try skull crushers (see page 81).

HOW CAN I PREVENT NECK PAIN WITH CRUNCHES?

Initiate the movement from your core rather than leading with your head. Keep a space between your chin and chest and try not to pull on your neck.

*DO YOU STRUGGLE
TO HOLD A PLANK
POSITION?*

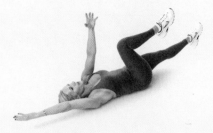

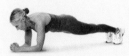

Try an alternative for
your core, such as dead
bugs (see page 56).

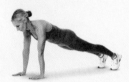

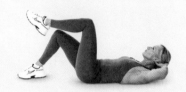

Or try toe taps (see
page 61), which are
great options for
strengthening the
deep core muscles.

*DO YOUR KNEES
HURT WHEN YOU
SQUAT OR LUNGE?*

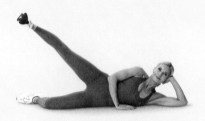

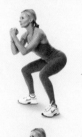

There are lots of
alternatives for
strengthening your
legs. Try side-lying leg
raises (or standing, see
page 71) and add a band
for extra resistance.

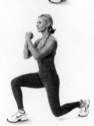

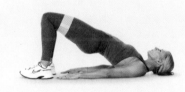

Or glute bridges (see
page 55) are also a
great alternative.

*MY BACK HURTS
WHEN I'M DOING MY
BENT-OVER ROWS*

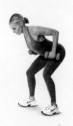

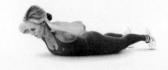

Try dorsal raises on
the mat (see page 58),
ensuring you do not
come up too high with
the upper body.

RECIPES TO
NOURISH

IN THE
KITCHEN

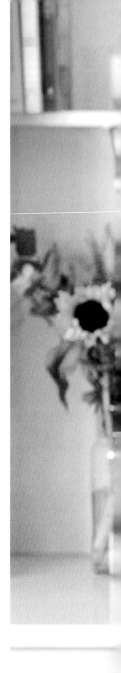

I really hope you're enjoying your six-week plan. However, it wouldn't be complete without sharing my favorite recipes with you, food that I love and that you can easily make at home.

Nourishing ourselves properly and making sure we enjoy our food is essential at any stage in our lives. It is also so important to fuel our bodies with the right foods to maintain healthy habits.

Combining the exercises and recipes in this six-week plan gives me the chance to show you how this can be achieved at home. It is so easy to fall into negative food patterns where we consider exercise as a way of burning off our food intake or earning the right to eat whatever we want post-workout. Instead, I would like to share ideas about how healthy eating can reframe our thinking and make food exciting. Uncoupling diet and exercise and instead focusing on eating and training for optimal health and function is, I believe, where there are the biggest wins for our health and happiness long-term.

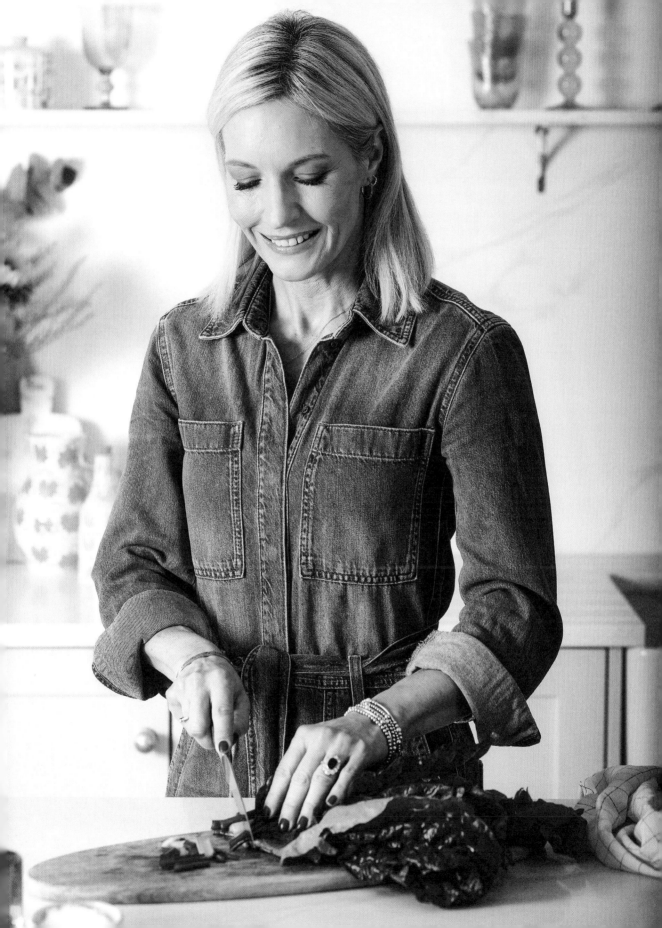

PLAN IT

I've included four examples of a daily meal plan, to show how the right balance of nutrients can come together to keep you satisfied. You'll notice that each recipe includes a breakdown of carbs, protein, and fiber, because I believe these are the areas worth focusing on. My recipes also contain sources of healthy fats, although I haven't listed the amount because calculating our fat intake in a day isn't necessary when we look at the balance of our meals as a whole. Some recipes have more carbohydrate in them than others—this is to be expected, as some vegetables, dairy, lentils, pulses, fruit, and sauce ingredients will all contribute to our carb intake. I try to ensure I get at least a couple of servings of whole grains every day because this helps to protect my cardiovascular health. You'll find whole grain serves in main meals as well as snacks. Finally, you'll see these combinations provide a great intake of fiber to help you to hit the recommended 30g a day, for improved gut health and diversity. These meal plans are designed to provide some inspiration, but are also flexible. Don't forget that not all snacks and desserts need to involve prep or fit certain criteria—feel free to add in your own choices, too. For me, it might be a piece of fruit, handful of nuts, or a couple of cookies, for example.

I find when my meals are well balanced, my snacks and desserts slot more in tune with my needs and vary day to day. Savor your food and weave in my golden fundamentals (see page 25) and you can't go wrong.

MEAL PLAN SUGGESTIONS				
BREAKFAST	Banana Granola (p. 153)	Better Avocado Toast (p. 156)	Coconut Cardamom Overnight Oats (p. 152)	Herb Omelet with Tomato & Bell Pepper Salad (p. 161)
SNACK	A snack of your choice	My Tracker Bars (p. 214)	Mocha Hazelnut Energy Bite (p. 213)	A snack of your choice
LUNCH	Greek Salad with Lemon & Oregano Shrimp (p. 164)	Chicken & Mushroom Pot Pie (p. 186)	Hot Honey Halloumi Salad (p. 166)	Moroccan Spiced Vegetables with Preserved Lemon Yogurt (p. 182)
DINNER	Zucchini & Spicy Sausage Pasta (p. 190)	Mustard Beany Salad Jar (p. 179)	Roasted Sea Bream with Greens & Tomato Salsa Verde (p. 207)	Miso Gyoza Soup (p. 176)
DESSERT	Girlled Tropical Fruit Salad (p. 228)	A dessert of your choice	A dessert of your choice	Date Caramel Chia Puddings (p. 225)

RECIPE KEY

I've marked the following recipes with these symbols to show you which provide the best sources of different nutrients.

PP — **PROTEIN PROVIDER**
Meals—provides at least 15–20g protein.
Snacks—provides at least 3g protein.
Desserts—provides at least 5g protein.

DW — **DIVERSITY WINNER**
Contains at least three different plant-based foods.

BS — **BONE SUPPORTER**
Contains dairy or plant-based calcium sources, such as canned fish, like sardines or tuna (including bones), calcium-set tofu, broccoli, kale, cabbage, sesame seeds and tahini, pulses, or nuts.

O3 — **OMEGA-3 GOODNESS**
Contains either oily fish or nuts or seeds, e.g. walnuts, flaxseeds, and chia seeds.

WG — **WHOLE GRAIN**
A source of whole grain so contributes toward daily recommendations.

LG — **LEAFY GREEN HIT**
Provides good essential minerals, e.g., iron or magnesium.

High-Protein Banana Pancakes

PP

DW

BS

WG

These pancakes sneak in cottage cheese for an extra hit of protein, but you can substitute Greek yogurt instead.

Serves 3 | Total time: 20 minutes

1 banana, plus extra slices to serve

2 eggs

5½oz (150g) cottage cheese

1 cup (100g) rolled oats

½ cup (125ml) soy milk or milk of your choice

½ tsp vanilla extract

¼ tsp ground cinnamon

½ tbsp honey or maple syrup, plus extra to serve

1 tsp baking powder

pinch of salt

1 tbsp butter

handful of pecans, coarsely chopped, to serve

Add the banana, eggs, cottage cheese, oats, milk, vanilla, cinnamon, maple syrup, baking powder, and salt to a blender and pulse until combined.

Heat a nonstick skillet on medium heat, then add a little bit of the butter, brushing it around with the back of your spoon.

Fry the pancakes in batches, allowing them to cook for 1–2 minutes on each side until golden and puffy. Add more butter to the pan for frying as needed. You should be able to make nine pancakes in total.

Serve with extra banana slices, chopped pecans, and a little drizzle of honey or maple syrup.

Protein | 17g/portion
Carbohydrate | 35g/portion
Fiber | 4.5g/portion

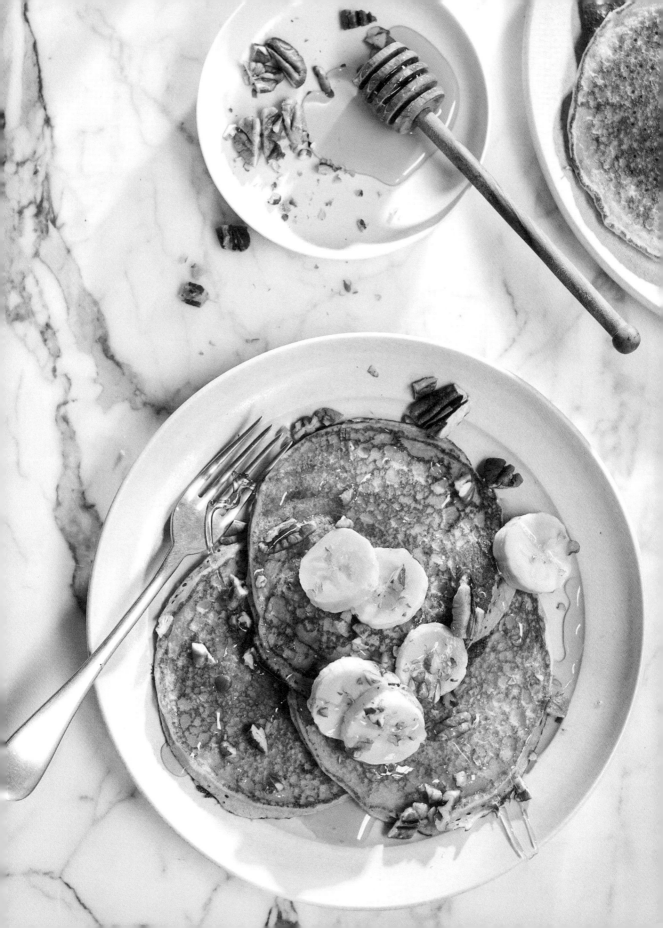

Raspberry Baked Oats with Ricotta

PP
DW
BS
WG

These baked oats can be enjoyed warm or sliced up and eaten like bars—amazing for an on-the-go breakfast.

Serves 4 | Total time: 35 minutes

2 bananas

2 cups (200g) rolled oats

2 eggs, beaten

1¾ cups (400ml) milk of your choice (soy is a good option for extra protein)

1 tsp vanilla extract

1 tsp baking powder

5½oz (150g) raspberries

½ cup (125g) ricotta

2 tbsp smooth almond butter

honey or maple syrup, to serve (optional)

Preheat the oven to 350°F (180°C).

Add the bananas to a mixing bowl and mash with a fork, then add the oats, eggs, milk, vanilla, and baking powder and mix well to combine.

Transfer to an 8 x 9in (20 x 25cm) dish and spread out evenly. Place the raspberries all over and then add dollops of the ricotta.

Transfer to the oven and bake for 30 minutes.

Remove from the oven and drizzle over the almond butter. Serve with a little honey or maple syrup, if desired.

Protein | 22g/portion
Carbohydrate | 46g/portion
Fiber | 7.3g/portion

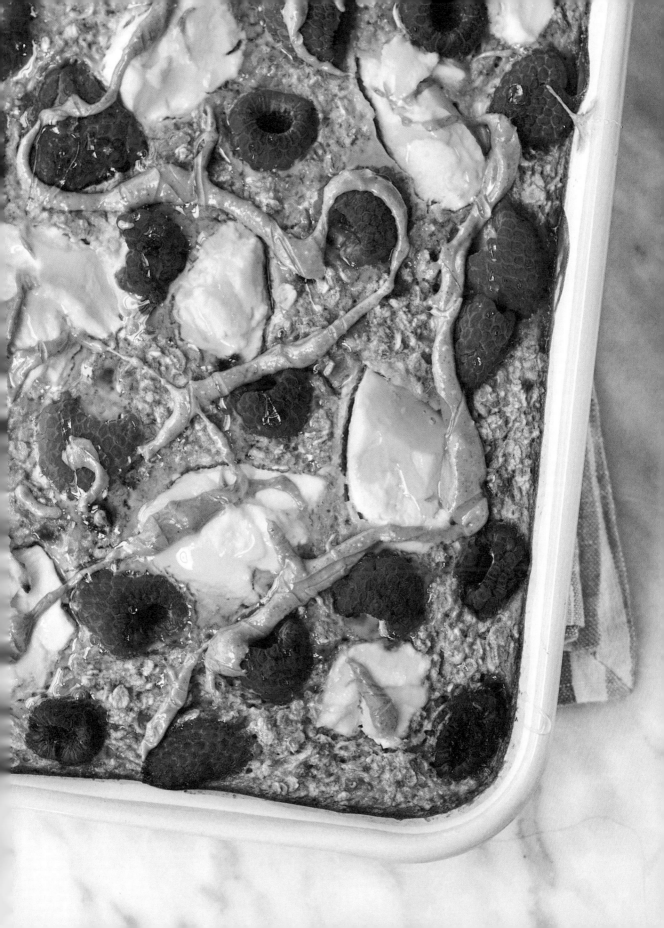

Coconut Cardamom Overnight Oats

BS
DW
O3
WG

These overnight oats are a great breakfast to prep ahead of time.

Serves 1 | Total time: 20 minutes, plus overnight chiling

5½oz (150g) frozen berries (I used blackberries, strawberries, and raspberries)

½ tsp vanilla extract

½ cup (50g) rolled oats

½ cup (120ml) soy milk

½ cup (50g) coconut yogurt or vegan yogurt of your choice

1 tbsp chia seeds

1 tsp ground cinnamon

½ tsp ground cardamom

TO SERVE (optional)

nut butter of your choice

sliced banana

Add the berries to a small saucepan and cook on medium heat for 10–15 minutes, until the mixture becomes a compote. Stir in the vanilla and let cool.

Mix the oats and soy milk together, then stir in the yogurt, chia seeds, cinnamon, and cardamom.

Spoon the oats and berry compote into a jar, alternating between the two to create nice layers. Transfer to the fridge until the next day.

Finish by topping with your favorite nut butter and sliced banana, if you like. Enjoy!

NOTE: If you'd prefer to use a milk with less protein than soy, you can add a scoop of protein powder of your choice, if desired.

Protein | 13g/portion
Carbohydrate | 46g/portion
Fiber | 18g/portion

Banana Granola

PP
DW
WG

This no-sugar granola is an amazing way to get plant diversity into your mornings—use whatever nuts and seeds you have on hand and switch it up the next time you make the recipe. The sweetness comes from the mashed bananas. This is also an oil-free granola, as I use egg white to bind the ingredients together—it makes them crisp and crunchy clusters, while adding a little extra protein too! Serve with yogurt and berries, drizzled with honey, if you like.

Serves 8–10 portions | Total time: 40 minutes

2 ripe bananas

2½ cups (250g) rolled oats

7oz (200g) mixed nuts (I used cashews, almonds, and walnuts), coarsely chopped

5½oz (150g) mixed seeds (I used linseed, sunflower, and pumpkin)

1 tbsp ground cinnamon

1 tsp vanilla extract

2 egg whites

2½oz (75g) dried cranberries

flaky sea salt

Preheat the oven to 325°F (160°C).

Put the bananas into a large mixing bowl and mash with a fork. Add the oats, nuts, seeds, cinnamon, vanilla, and a generous pinch of flaky sea salt. Mix well to combine.

In a separate bowl, whisk the egg whites until frothy, then pour into the granola mix and stir well to coat.

Transfer to a large baking sheet, spreading the mixture out evenly. Bake for 30 minutes, stirring halfway through.

Remove from the oven and stir in the dried cranberries. Store in a sealed container for up to 2 weeks.

Protein | 16g/portion
Carbohydrate | 35g/portion
Fiber | 5.7g/portion

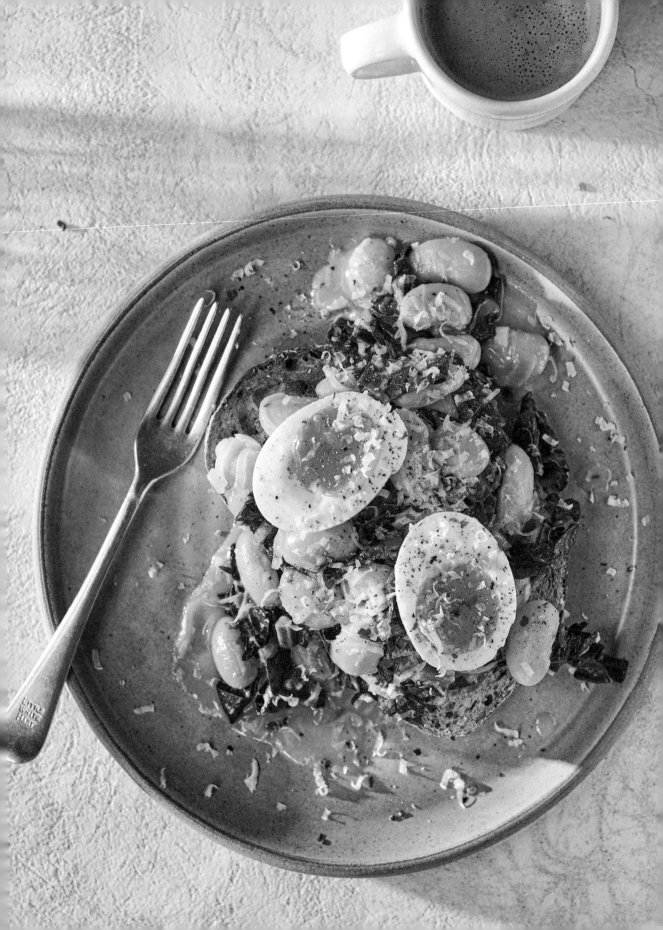

Cheesy Beans on Toast with Tuscan Kale

These are a fantastic source of protein. Super quick to prepare, they are way more nutritious than sugary beans from a can.

Serves 2 | Total time: 25 minutes

1 tbsp extra virgin olive oil

2 shallots, thinly sliced

2 garlic cloves, grated

pinch of chili flakes

1½ cans (570g) of butter beans (lima beans), plus their liquid

5½oz (150g) Tuscan kale, tough stems removed and coarsely chopped

juice of ½ lemon

1¼oz (40g) Parmesan cheese, grated

2 eggs (optional)

2 slices of seeded whole-grain bread of your choice

Set a large skillet on medium heat and add the olive oil and shallots. Sauté for 8 minutes until softened, then add the garlic and chili flakes and cook for another 2 minutes.

Add the butter beans to the pan along with their liquid and stir to combine.

Add the Tuscan kale to the pan and squeeze the lemon juice over the top. Cover with a lid and cook for 5 minutes to wilt the greens.

Remove the lid and stir in most of the Parmesan.

If you like, you can also add a boiled egg. Add one egg per person to a small pan of boiling water and cook for 6½ minutes for a jammy egg. Refresh under cold water. Toast the bread.

Serve the beans on top of the toast, topped with an egg, if using. Finish with the remaining Parmesan and an extra pinch of chili flakes, if you like.

Hot tip

These would be easy to make vegan, just swap the Parmesan for nutritional yeast or your favorite vegan cheese, and serve without eggs.

Protein | 29g/portion
Carbohydrate | 57g/portion
Fiber | 23g/portion

Better Avocado Toast

PP

DW

O3

I absolutely adore avocado—as you can see, it features quite a lot in the book! I wanted to find a way of adding extra protein and greens at breakfast to balance out healthy fats. Blending the avocado with edamame makes the avocado go further, too, saving you money and increasing the nutritional value overall.

Serves 2 | Total time: 20 minutes

5½oz (150g) cherry tomatoes

1 tsp extra virgin olive oil

1 avocado

3½oz (100g) edamame

juice of 1 lemon

2 slices of seeded sourdough or high-protein bread

3½oz (100g) spinach

1½ tbsp white wine vinegar

2 eggs

2 tbsp mixed seeds (I used sunflower, pumpkin, linseed, and sesame)

salt and freshly ground black pepper

Drizzle the cherry tomatoes with the olive oil and place in an air fryer at 350°F (180°C) for 12 minutes. Alternatively, you can roast in the oven at 350°F (180°C) for 16–18 minutes.

In the meantime, blend the avocado and edamame together with the lemon juice and a generous sprinkle of salt and pepper in a food processor, or mash by hand for a chunkier result.

Pop the sourdough in the toaster and toast to your liking.

Put the spinach in a small saucepan with a splash of water and cook for 1–2 minutes until wilted. Remove from the pan and set aside.

Fill the pan with water and bring to a boil. Add the white wine vinegar, then reduce the heat to low. Crack the eggs directly into the water, staying very close to the surface. Allow the eggs to poach for 2–3 minutes—use a slotted spoon to poke the egg to see when the white is set but the yolk is still runny.

Spread the avocado on the toast and top with two eggs and a sprinkling of seeds. Serve with the wilted spinach and roasted cherry tomatoes. Enjoy.

Protein | 17g/portion
Carbohydrate | 27g/portion
Fiber | 7.4g/portion

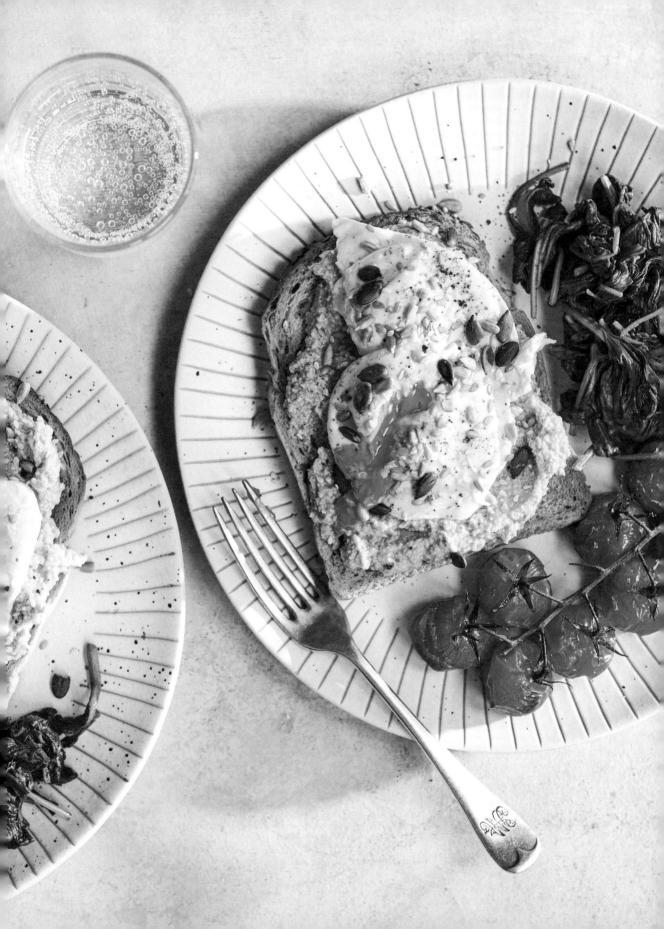

Kimchi & Avocado Toast

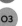

A super-quick breakfast full of flavor. Kimchi, tahini, and avocado are made for each other. Kimchi is an example of a fermented food which also supports our gut bacteria to thrive.

Serves 1 | Total time: 5 minutes

1 slice of rye bread

½ avocado, sliced

1¾oz (50g) kimchi

1 radish, thinly sliced

1 tbsp tahini

1 tbsp mixed seeds (I used sunflower, pumpkin, linseed, and sesame)

small handful of herb of your choice, leaves picked

Toast the rye bread.

Top with the sliced avocado, kimchi, and, finally, the sliced radish. Drizzle over the tahini, then sprinkle over the seeds. Finish with the herbs and dig in!

Protein | 14g/portion
Carbohydrate | 35g/portion
Fiber | 8.4g/portion

Breakfast Quesadilla

This cheesy, softly scrambled egg filling inside a whole-grain wrap is one of the best starts to the day—I love mine covered in hot sauce.

Serves 2 | Total time: 20 minutes

1 tbsp butter or olive oil

2 green onions, finely sliced

1 green bell pepper, seeded and finely diced

1 green chili, finely chopped

4 eggs

2 whole-grain tortilla wraps

4 slices of cheese of your choice (I like Gouda, Cheddar, or mozzarella cheese)

handful of cilantro, chopped

salt and freshly ground black pepper

hot sauce, to serve

Add the butter to a nonstick skillet (big enough for your wraps).

Add the green onions, green bell pepper, and chili and sauté on medium heat for 1–2 minutes, until sizzling and fragrant.

Beat the eggs in a bowl with a pinch of salt and pepper, then pour onto the cooking veggies. Scramble for 2–3 minutes until the eggs have just set and the egg still looks nice and glossy.

With a spatula, set the eggs aside, then place one wrap on the bottom of the pan. Spoon the eggs onto the wrap, top with the cheese and cilantro, then place the other wrap on top.

Fry for 1–2 minutes, then carefully flip the quesadilla over (using a plate if you need to, to slide it back into the pan).

Remove from the pan, cut into wedges, and drizzle with hot sauce.

Protein | 27g/portion
Carbohydrate | 31g/portion
Fiber | 7.8g/portion

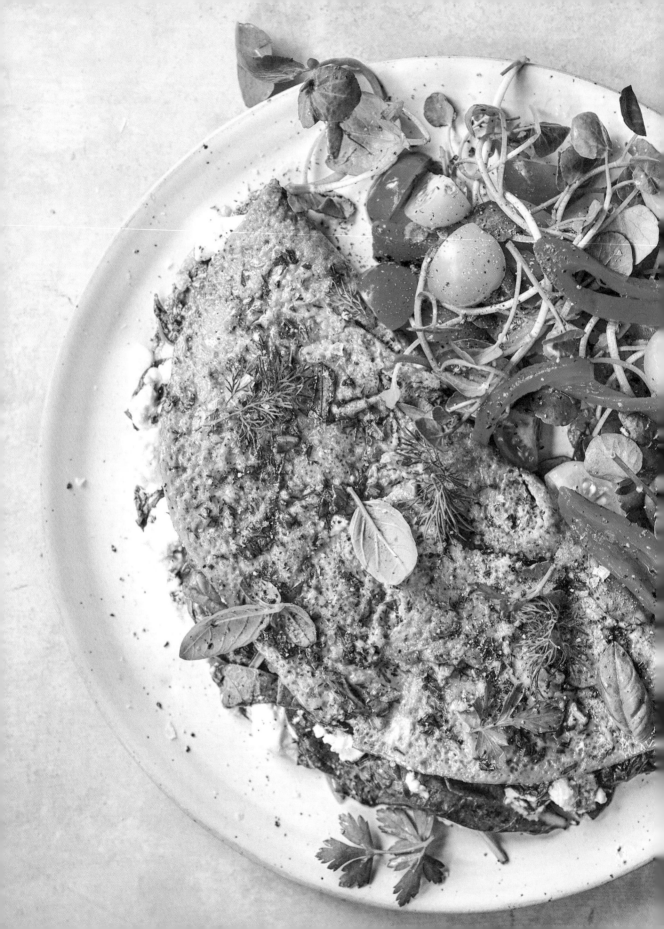

Herb Omelet with Tomato & Bell Pepper Salad

A vibrant green kick-start to your morning—a perfect meal for brunch too.

Serves 1 | Total time: 10 minutes

3 large eggs

1oz (30g) mixed herbs, finely chopped (I like basil, parsley, and dill, but use whatever soft herbs you have), plus extra to garnish

low-calorie oil spray

1 roasted red bell pepper, thinly sliced

handful of cherry tomatoes, quartered

handful of watercress

1oz (30g) baby spinach

1oz (25g) feta

salt and freshly ground black pepper

In a small bowl, lightly beat the eggs. Add the herbs and a pinch of salt, then stir to combine.

Heat a nonstick skillet on medium heat and add some oil spray.

Pour in the egg mixture and tilt the pan to ensure it spreads evenly. Let it cook undisturbed for 30 seconds, then use a spatula to move the mixture around a little, tilting again to spread the uncooked egg. Cook for another 1–2 minutes, until the egg is almost set.

Mix the red bell pepper, tomatoes, and watercress in a small bowl and season well.

Place the spinach and feta across one half of the omelet, then gently lift the other half and fold it over the filling.

Slide the omelet onto a plate and garnish with the extra herbs, and the salad alongside.

Protein | 18g/portion
Carbohydrate | 11g/portion
Fiber | 3.9g/portion

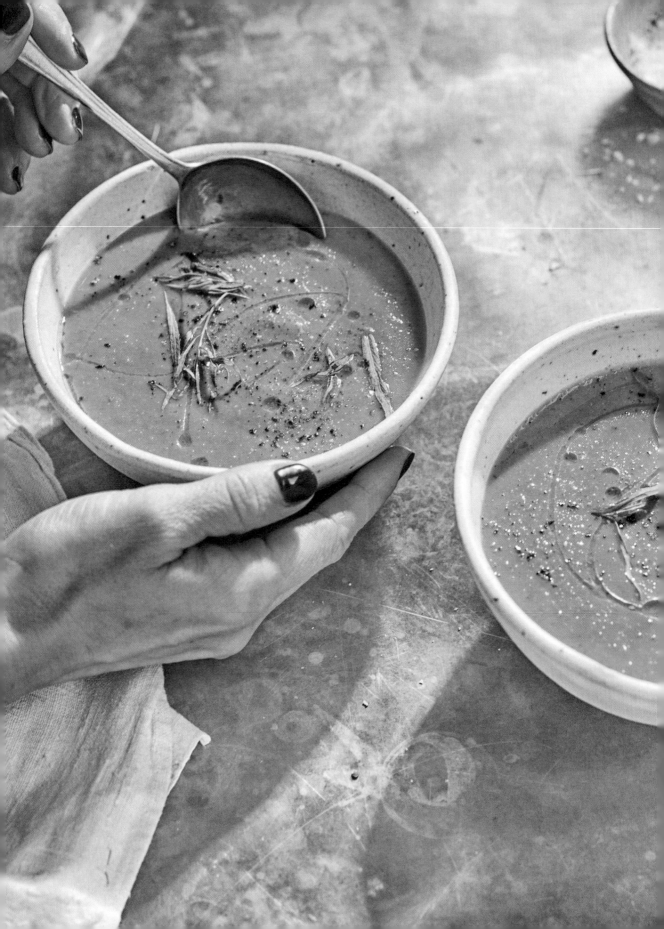

Tomato & Tarragon Soup

A soup is an incredible meal to prep for the week—nourishing, easy, and quick. This soup sneaks in some red lentils for extra nutrients and features my favorite flavor combination—tomatoes and tarragon. Heaven with a flatbread or grilled cheese!

Serves 4 | Total time: 1 hour

2lb 4oz (1kg) tomatoes

1 garlic bulb, halved

2 large shallots, peeled and halved

1 tbsp extra virgin olive oil, plus extra to serve

10oz (300g) split red lentils

5 cups (1.2 liters) vegetable stock

1 tbsp red wine vinegar

1oz (25g) fresh tarragon, tough stems removed

salt and freshly ground black pepper

Preheat the oven to 425°F (220°C).

Arrange the whole tomatoes, halved garlic bulb, and shallots on a baking sheet and drizzle with the olive oil.

Roast for 30–40 minutes until slightly charred and soft.

In the meantime, add the red lentils and stock to a large saucepan and simmer for 10–15 minutes, until the lentils are soft. Turn off the heat and set aside.

When the tomatoes are ready, squeeze the soft garlic cloves out of their papery skins and discard the skins. Add everything to the large saucepan, including the vinegar and tarragon (reserving some leaves for a garnish), and use a stick blender to puree until smooth. Feel free to add more boiling water to get the consistency you like.

Season with more red wine vinegar and salt and pepper to taste, swirl in a little extra virgin olive oil, and top with the reserved tarragon leaves.

Hot tip

This soup can be frozen for up to 3 months.

Protein | 22g/portion
Carbohydrate | 45g/portion
Fiber | 16g/portion

Greek Salad with Lemon & Oregano Shrimp

PP
DW
BS

I am a huge fan of a Greek salad, but it typically lacks in protein. Here, I've added one of my favorite ingredients—shrimp—but you can swap the shrimp for chicken, steak, or even a couple of boiled eggs. This salad is particularly good with a whole-grain pita.

Serves 2 | Total time: 25 minutes

1 lemon

a few sprigs of oregano, finely chopped

2 garlic cloves, minced

2 tbsp extra virgin olive oil

½ red onion, thinly sliced

2 tbsp red wine vinegar

½ tsp dried oregano

7oz (200g) raw peeled jumbo shrimp

9oz (250g) cherry tomatoes, halved

½ cucumber, diced

1 green bell pepper, seeded and diced

4oz (120g) Kalamata olives

⅓ cup (40g) feta, crumbled

salt and freshly ground black pepper

Start by zesting the lemon and squeezing the juice of half into a small bowl. Add the oregano, garlic, and 1 tablespoon of the extra virgin olive oil. Season with salt and pepper and set aside.

Then, in a large bowl, add the red onion slices and the remaining lemon juice, along with the remaining extra virgin olive oil, the red wine vinegar, and dried oregano. Add a big pinch of salt, mix well, and set aside.

Get a skillet nice and hot on high heat, then dry-fry the shrimp to encourage them to get a good, slightly charred color on them. When they are pink and cooked through, add the lemon, garlic, and oregano mixture and toss well to coat with the heat off.

Add the tomatoes, cucumber, bell pepper, and olives to the bowl with the red onion, which should be slightly pickled and less intense now. Toss well to combine.

Top with the shrimp and crumbled feta and enjoy.

Protein | 26g/portion
Carbohydrate | 13g/portion
Fiber | 6.8g/portion

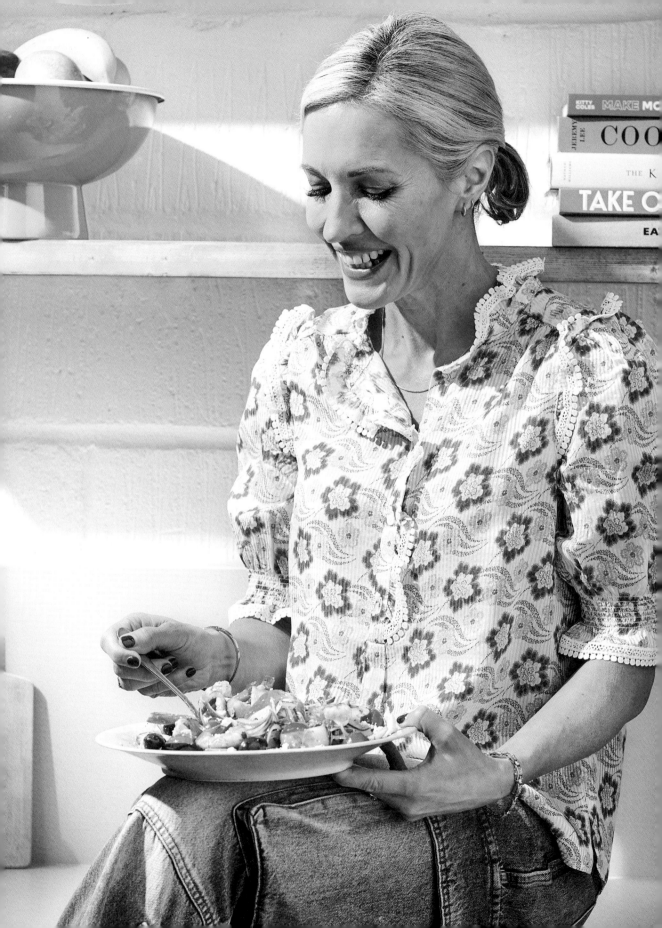

Hot Honey Halloumi Salad

PP

DW

BS

LG

I am a HUGE fan of halloumi, especially during the summer. With the spicy and sweet honey, it is just amazing! If you can't get your hands on it, just stir a pinch of chili flakes into some honey.

Serves 4 | Total time: 20 minutes

¼ red cabbage, shredded

½ Napa cabbage, shredded

2 small carrots, shredded

large handful of dill, finely chopped

½ bunch of chives

⅔ cup (150g) Greek yogurt

3½ tbsp white wine vinegar

½ tbsp extra virgin olive oil

9oz (250g) block of halloumi cheese, sliced

1 x 15oz (425g) can of chickpeas, drained and rinsed

3 tbsp hot honey

1 red chili, finely sliced (optional)

salt and freshly ground black pepper

Toss the two types of cabbage and carrot together with most of the dill and chives, saving some for the garnish. Stir in the yogurt and white wine vinegar and season to taste. Set aside.

Add the olive oil to a skillet on medium heat and sear the halloumi for 1–2 minutes on each side until golden. Add the chickpeas to warm through, then drizzle with hot honey.

Serve the halloumi and chickpeas on top of the slaw with the reserved herbs and red chili, if using.

Protein | 28g/portion
Carbohydrate | 37g/portion
Fiber | 10g/portion

Hot Buffalo Chicken Wrap

This wrap is HOT stuff, and unbelievably delicious. I've made a quick yogurt dip to help cool off the spice, but that's totally optional.

Makes 2 | Total time: 15 minutes

2 cooked skinless chicken breasts, shredded

½ cup (100g) Greek yogurt

4 tbsp buffalo sauce

1 large celery rib, finely diced

2 whole-grain tortilla wraps

2oz (60g) spinach

⅓ cup (40g) grated mozzarella cheese

small handful of pickles (optional)

salt and freshly ground black pepper

FOR THE YOGURT DIP (optional)

¾ cup (175g) kefir or Greek yogurt

½ tsp garlic powder

bunch of chives

juice of ½ lemon

1 tbsp nutritional yeast

In a small bowl, mix the shredded chicken with the yogurt, buffalo sauce, and celery. Ensure everything is evenly coated and season generously to taste. Set aside.

In another small bowl, mix together all the ingredients for the yogurt dip, if using.

Pile half of the filling on to each tortilla wrap and top with half of the spinach and half of the mozzarella. Add the pickles, if using. Tuck both opposite sides of the wrap over the filling, then roll from the bottom up to secure—you need to hold on tightly to keep all the filling inside.

Transfer the wraps to a dry skillet and toast for 1–2 minutes on each side until golden and crisp.

Serve with the yogurt dip, if using, and enjoy.

Protein | 59g/portion
Carbohydrate | 35g/portion
Fiber | 9.2g/portion

Watermelon Poke Bowl

PP

DW
BS

Once you've tried this marinated watermelon, you'll never go back to tuna in a poke bowl—it absorbs the flavors well and is so refreshing yet punchy to eat. I've added extra protein to this bowl by making a sriracha "mayo" that blends sriracha and silken tofu.

Serves 3 | Total time: 30 minutes

10oz (300g) watermelon, peeled and diced

4 tbsp light soy sauce

1 tbsp rice vinegar

1 tsp sesame oil

1 garlic clove, grated

2in (5cm) piece of fresh ginger, grated

5½oz (150g) silken tofu

2 tbsp sriracha

1 x 9oz (250g) microwaveable pouch of sticky rice

5½oz (150g) edamame

2 small carrots, julienned

1 avocado, diced

5½oz (150g) mango, diced

8 radishes, thinly sliced

¼ cucumber, thinly sliced

1 tbsp sesame seeds

small handful of cilantro leaves

Mix together the watermelon cubes, soy sauce, vinegar, sesame oil, garlic, and ginger. Set aside to marinate for 20 minutes.

Blend together the silken tofu and sriracha in a small blender or using a handheld blender. Set aside.

Heat the rice in the microwave according to the package instructions, then divide between two bowls.

Arrange the vegetables in ingredient sections to give a colorful array, then divide the watermelon among the bowls, making sure to drizzle over plenty of the marinade on the rice.

Pour over the sriracha "mayo" and sprinkle on the sesame seeds and cilantro leaves. Enjoy.

Protein | 15g/portion
Carbohydrate | 50g/portion
Fiber | 8.4g/portion

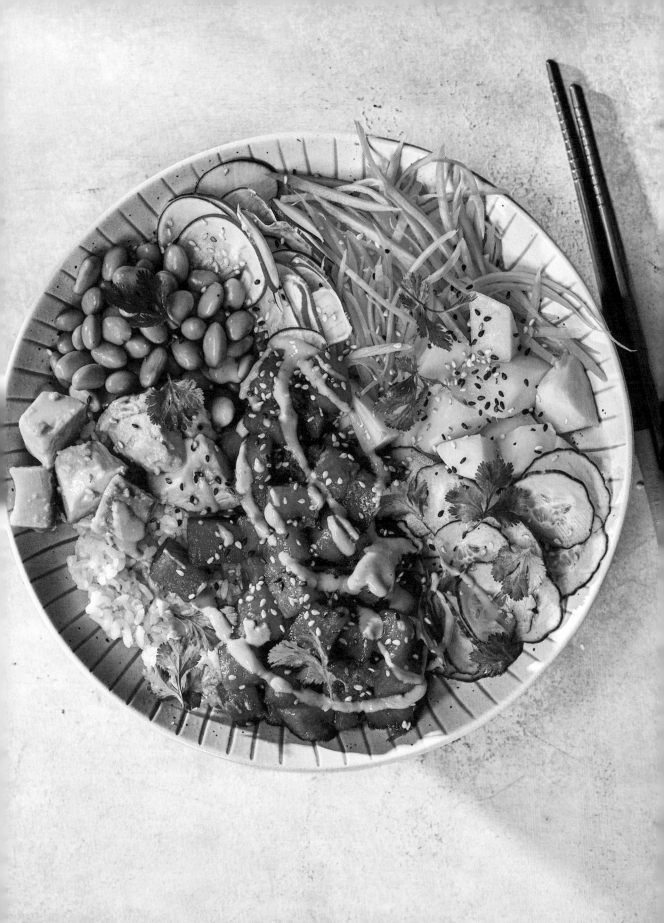

Shrimp Summer Rolls with Peanut Dipping Sauce

The most beautiful lunch! Not only do these rolls look incredible, but they taste so good and are also very satisfying to make.

Serves 1 | Total time: 20 minutes

4 rice paper wrappers

5½oz (150g) cooked jumbo shrimp

1 small carrot, julienned

¼ red cabbage, very thinly sliced

½ head Baby Gem or butter lettuce, shredded

small bunch of mint, leaves picked

small bunch of cilantro

sesame seeds, to garnish

FOR THE PEANUT DIPPING SAUCE

1 tbsp smooth peanut butter

½ tsp light soy sauce

¼ tsp honey

juice of ½ lime, to taste

Fill a large, high-sided pan with some water. Working one at a time, soak a rice paper sheet until it softens slightly and becomes pliable.

Lay the rice paper wrapper on a cutting board. Place three shrimp along the center, then top with the carrot, cabbage, and lettuce, finishing with the mint leaves and cilantro sprigs. Lift the side farthest from you over the filling, then fold in the sides as tightly as you can—try to also be delicate so you don't tear the rice paper!

Roll the filling toward you once, then lift the rice paper edge closest to you over the filling to seal.

Repeat with the remaining ingredients to make four summer rolls in total.

Add the peanut butter, soy sauce, honey, and lime juice to a small bowl and mix. Loosen with a splash of boiling water to make the sauce a dipping consistency.

Serve the summer rolls sprinkled with sesame seeds and the sauce alongside for dipping.

Protein | 30g/portion
Carbohydrate | 49g/portion
Fiber | 11g/portion

Tuna Crunch Wrap

*This crunchy and delicious wrap is an all-time favorite
in my house, and so quick to put together.*

Serves 2 | Total time: 20 minutes

*5oz (145g) can of tuna in
water, drained*

¼ cup (40g) Greek yogurt

1 tsp adobo sauce

juice of ½ lime

1 green onion, thinly sliced

2 medium whole-grain tortillas

*¼ cup (30g) Cheddar cheese,
grated*

*1 roasted red bell pepper,
sliced*

large handful of watercress

*small handful of whole-grain
tortilla chips*

flaky sea salt

Add the tuna, yogurt, adobo, and lime juice to a bowl. Mix well,
then stir in the green onion and a pinch of salt.

Assemble your wrap. Lay one of the tortillas on a cutting board
and sprinkle the Cheddar cheese over the center. Spoon the tuna
mixture over the cheese, then top with the red bell pepper,
followed by the watercress, and finishing with the tortilla chips.

Cut the other tortilla into a smaller circle that neatly covers the
filling and place it on top. Fold up the edges of the first tortilla in a
fan pattern, overlapping the edges of the wrap to safely enclose
the filling inside.

Set a skillet on medium heat and gently transfer the wrap into the
pan, seal-side down. Cook for 5–10 minutes, flipping once until the
folded side is well sealed and the wrap is nicely browned.

Cut in half and enjoy!

Protein | 25g/portion
Carbohydrate | 36g/portion
Fiber | 6.8g/portion

Hot Smoked Salmon Niçoise

PP
DW
O3

Hot smoked salmon is a good oily fish, which is a wonderful addition to our diets. This is an amazing twist on the classic tuna Niçoise.

Serves 2 | Total time: 25 minutes

*7oz (200g) baby or
new potatoes*

*5½oz (150g) green beans,
trimmed*

3 eggs

1¼oz (40g) Kalamata olives

*3½oz (100g) mixed salad
leaves*

*5½oz (150g) cherry tomatoes,
halved*

2 tbsp capers (optional)

*5½oz (150g) hot smoked
salmon*

*salt and freshly ground
black pepper*

FOR THE DRESSING

4 anchovy fillets

2 tsp Dijon mustard

2 tbsp red wine vinegar

3 tbsp extra virgin olive oil

Bring a large pot of salted water to a boil. Add the potatoes, green beans, and eggs. Remove the green beans after 3 minutes, the eggs after 7 minutes, and the potatoes after 15 minutes, or tender when pierced with a paring knife. Run the eggs under cold water, crack the shells and peel, then quarter the eggs. Halve the potatoes if they are large.

In the meantime, finely chop the anchovies and whisk together all of the remaining dressing ingredients. Season to taste.

Put the rest of the salad ingredients in a bowl with the olives, salad, tomatoes, and capers, if using. Flake in large chunks of the salmon.

Drizzle with the dressing and season well with black pepper. Enjoy.

Protein | 38g/portion
Carbohydrate | 22g/portion
Fiber | 6.9g/portion

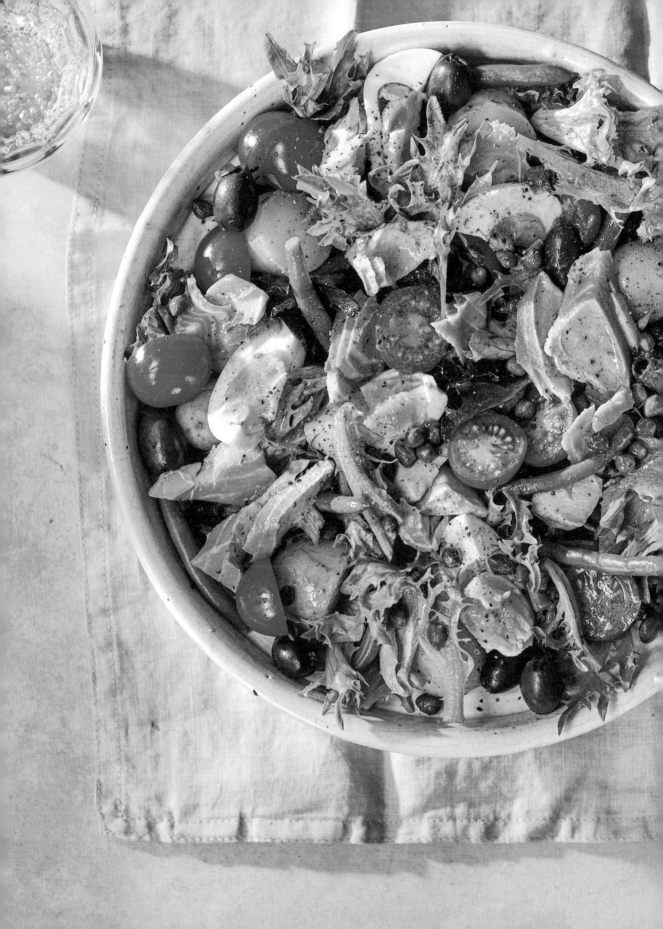

Thai Chicken Salad

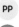

This shredded salad is incredibly fragrant and aromatic. I absolutely love using fresh lime leaves, and you can get them in most big supermarkets now—they really make such a difference to this dish. I use precooked chicken for ease, but feel free to cook your own if you like!

Serves 4 | Total time: 20 minutes

4 skinless chicken breasts, cooked

2 carrots, julienned

2 heads of Baby Gem or butter lettuce, shredded

4 green onions, thinly sliced

1 shallot, thinly sliced

1 lemongrass, tough stem removed and thinly sliced

4 fresh makrut lime leaves, shredded

3½oz (100g) edamame

3½oz (100g) frozen peas (see Note)

small bunch of cilantro

small bunch of mint, torn

handful of roasted peanuts, coarsely chopped

FOR THE DRESSING

juice of 3 limes

1 tbsp sesame oil

2 tbsp fish sauce

1 red chili, finely chopped

1 garlic clove, grated

Use two forks to shred the chicken breasts, then add to a large mixing bowl with the carrots, lettuce, green onions, shallot, lemongrass, lime leaves, edamame, peas, cilantro, and mint. Mix well to combine.

In a small bowl, mix all the dressing ingredients together.

Pour the dressing over the salad and toss together.

Serve the salad topped with the roasted peanuts.

NOTE: Using frozen peas here might sound a bit strange, but they'll defrost before you start eating!

Protein | 40g/portion
Carbohydrate | 9.9g/portion
Fiber | 6.6g/portion

LIGHTER BITES

Lentil, Sardine/Halloumi Power Bowl

It's totally up to you whether you opt for halloumi or sardines here—they both work beautifully in this flexitarian recipe.

Serves 2 | Total time: 20 minutes

½ red onion

2 lemons

7oz (200g) Tuscan kale, stems removed, finely shredded

3½oz (100g) asparagus spears, shaved

1 tbsp extra virgin olive oil, plus ½ tbsp extra if using halloumi cheese

1 avocado

bunch of chives

large handful of tarragon

1 tbsp Greek yogurt

9oz (250g) halloumi cheese OR 2 x 4½oz (125g) can of sardines

1 x 9oz (250g) pouch of cooked Puy lentils

2 roasted red bell peppers, thinly sliced

1¼oz (40g) pomegranate seeds

salt and freshly ground black pepper

In a small bowl, combine the red onion with the juice of 1 lemon, plus a big pinch of salt. Mix to start the pickling process and set aside.

Add the juice of the remaining lemon to a large bowl, toss in the Tuscan kale and asparagus shavings along with a tablespoon of extra virgin olive oil. Massage briefly for around 30 seconds and set aside.

Using a handheld blender, blend the avocado, chives, tarragon, yogurt, and approximately ⅓ cup (100ml) cold water to loosen.

Cook the halloumi in a skillet on high heat in the reserved half tablespoon of extra virgin olive oil for 1–2 minutes on each side until golden. Alternatively, open the cans of sardines.

Heat the Puy lentils in the microwave according to the package instructions.

Add the bell peppers, pomegranate seeds, and pickled onions to the bowl of kale and top with either the halloumi or sardines. Drizzle over the dressing and enjoy.

Protein | 50g/portion
Carbohydrate | 43g/portion
Fiber | 16g/portion

*if using sardines

Miso Gyoza Soup

PP
DW
BS
LG

This is an emergency freezer situation, so take all of the veggies here as a guide. The aim is to use up whatever fresh or frozen vegetables you have on hand—the main thing is to keep a stash of high-protein tofu gyoza in the freezer for whenever the craving strikes.

Serves 1 | Total time: 10 minutes

1 tbsp white miso paste

5 tofu gyoza

1 green onion, green and white parts separated, thinly sliced

1oz (30g) shiitake mushrooms

1 baby bok choy, cut into quarters

3½oz (100g) edamame

1 tsp light soy sauce

juice of ½ lime

chili crisp oil, to serve

Add the miso to a saucepan with 1½ cups (350ml) of boiling water. Set on medium heat and whisk to dissolve the miso.

Add the gyoza, whites of the green onion, and the mushrooms and cook for 4 minutes, adding the bok choy and edamame for the final 2 minutes.

Season the broth with the soy sauce and lime juice.

Serve in a big bowl with the sliced green onion tops and chili crisp oil.

Protein | 25g/portion
Carbohydrate | 42g/portion
Fiber | 12g/portion

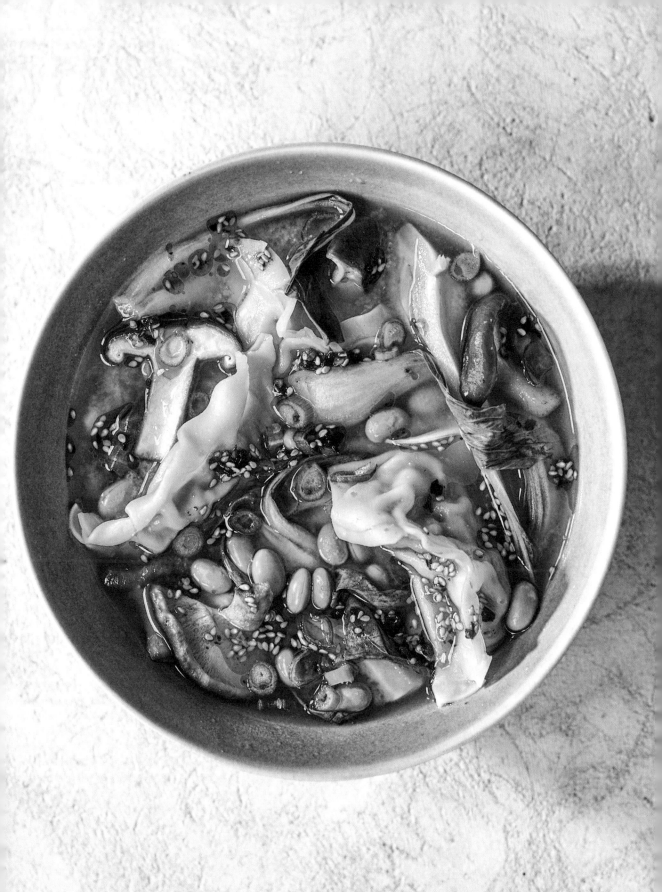

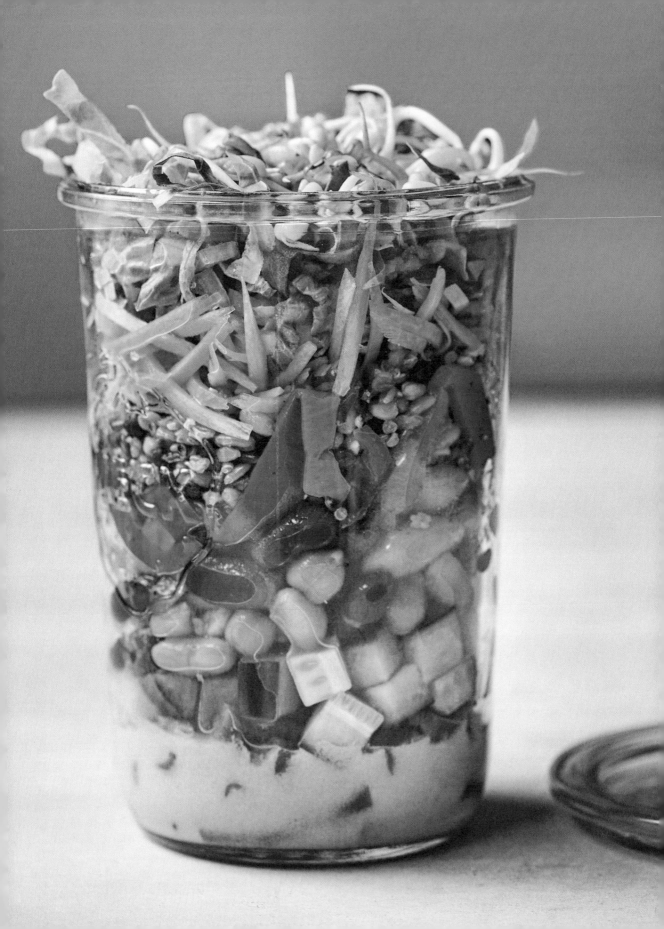

Mustardy Beany Salad Jar

This makes one large jar for two, or two smaller jars. It is ideal for meal prep, as you can pour the whole thing out onto a plate for a perfectly dressed salad, ready to go. Just look at those colors!

Serves 2 | Total time: 10 minutes

3½oz (100g) green beans, trimmed and cut into thirds

1 tbsp extra virgin olive oil

1 tbsp Dijon mustard

1 tbsp apple cider vinegar

½ garlic clove, minced

¼ cucumber, diced

½ x 14oz (400g) can of mixed beans

1 roasted red bell pepper, thinly sliced

½ x 9oz (250g) pouch of precooked mixed grains

1 carrot, grated

1 Baby Gem or butter lettuce, shredded

small handful of sprouts

2 tbsp mixed seeds (I used pumpkin, sunflower, linseed, and sesame)

salt

Blanch the green beans in boiling water for 3–4 minutes until cooked. Set aside to cool.

Mix the olive oil, mustard, apple cider vinegar, and garlic together with a pinch of salt.

Layer the salad in a large jar or plastic container, or two smaller jars if preferred. Start with the mustard dressing, followed by the green beans and cucumber. Next, add the mixed beans, followed by the sliced red bell pepper and mixed grains. Then add the grated carrot and lettuce, then the sprouts and, finally, the seeds.

When you're ready to eat, turn the jar out into a bowl, mix well, and enjoy.

Protein | 37g/portion
Carbohydrate | 102g/portion
Fiber | 29g/portion

Chicken & Nectarine Panzanella

PP

DW

BS

LG

This is one of those salads that I make on repeat all summer long.
It tastes the best with the ripest fresh produce you can find.

Serves 2 | Total time: 25 minutes

2 slices of seeded sourdough, cut into chunks

2 tbsp extra virgin olive oil

2 skin-on chicken breasts

1 shallot, thinly sliced into rounds

juice of ½ lemon

2 large vine tomatoes, cut into chunks

2 nectarines, cut into chunks

bunch of basil, leaves picked

1 tbsp red wine or sherry vinegar

2¾oz (80g) watercress

4½oz (125g) mozzarella di bufala bocconcini

salt

Preheat the oven to 350°F (180°C). Spread the sourdough chunks over a large baking sheet and toss with 1 tablespoon of the olive oil and a pinch of salt.

Heat a skillet on medium-high heat. Once hot, add the chicken breasts, skin-side down, and cook for 5 minutes until the skin is golden brown and crisp. Flip and cook on the other side for another 5 minutes, then transfer to the baking sheet with the croutons.

Transfer the chicken and croutons to the oven and bake for 15 minutes until the croutons are golden and the chicken is cooked through.

In the meantime, add the sliced shallots to a mixing bowl and squeeze in the lemon juice. Use your hands to mix them up, then add the tomatoes, nectarines, basil, vinegar, and the remaining olive oil. Season with a pinch of salt and toss together. Set aside to macerate.

When the chicken and croutons are cooked, remove from the oven. Slice the chicken into bite-sized chunks and add the croutons to the salad, also adding the watercress and mozzarella, tearing any large bocconcini.

Serve the salad with the sliced chicken on top and enjoy!

Protein | 56g/portion
Carbohydrate | 30g/portion
Fiber | 3.9g/portion

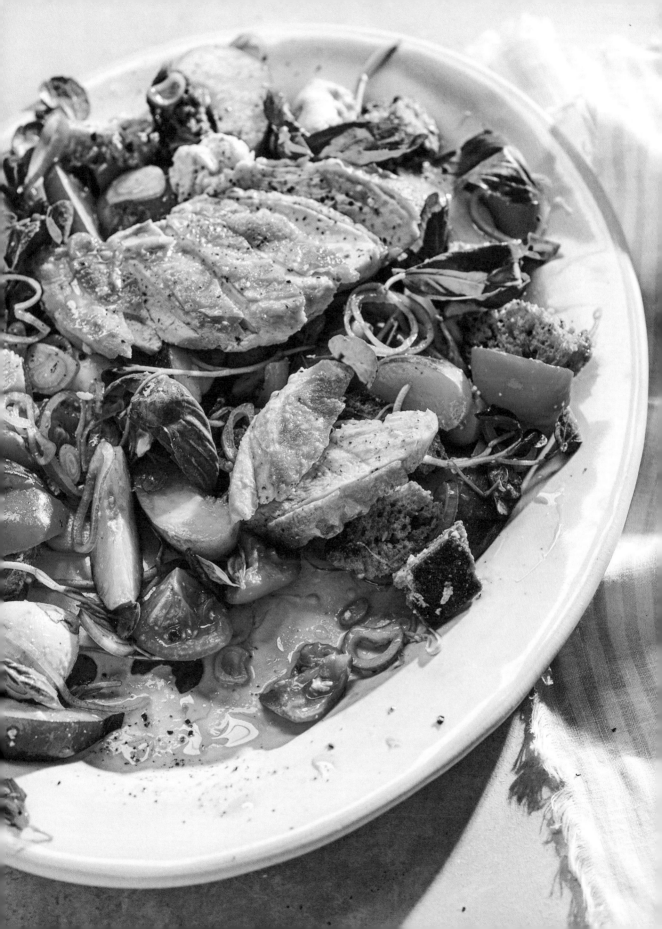

Moroccan Spiced Vegetables with Preserved Lemon Yogurt

A wonderful veggie-packed dinner that also can be prepared in advance.

PP
DW
BS
WG
LG

Serves 4 | Total time: 40 minutes

1 red onion, cut into wedges

1 cauliflower, torn into florets and leaves reserved

½ Napa cabbage, cut into thin wedges and leaves reserved

2 bell peppers of your choice, seeded and coarsely chopped

1½ x 15oz cans (570g) of chickpeas, drained

2 tbsp ras al hanout

2 x 9oz (250g) microwaveable pouches of quinoa

small bunch of parsley, finely chopped

sumac, to serve

FOR THE PRESERVED LEMON YOGURT

½ cup (120g) Greek yogurt

1 garlic clove, grated

2 preserved lemons

flaky sea salt

Preheat the oven to 400°F (200°C).

Add the red onion wedges, cauliflower florets and leaves, cabbage, bell peppers, and chickpeas to a large roasting pan. Sprinkle over the ras al hanout, then use your hands to mix the spice into the vegetables, distributing it as evenly as possible.

Transfer the vegetables to the oven and roast for 30 minutes until cooked and nicely browned.

In the meantime, loosen the yogurt with a couple of tablespoons of water and add the garlic. Cut the preserved lemons into quarters, then cut out the flesh and discard. Finely chop the peel and add this to the yogurt, along with a generous pinch of salt.

Cook the quinoa according to the package instructions.

Serve the veggies over a bed of quinoa, drizzling the yogurt on top. Finish with the finely chopped parsley and a pinch of sumac.

Protein | 28g/portion
Carbohydrate | 87g/portion
Fiber | 23g/portion

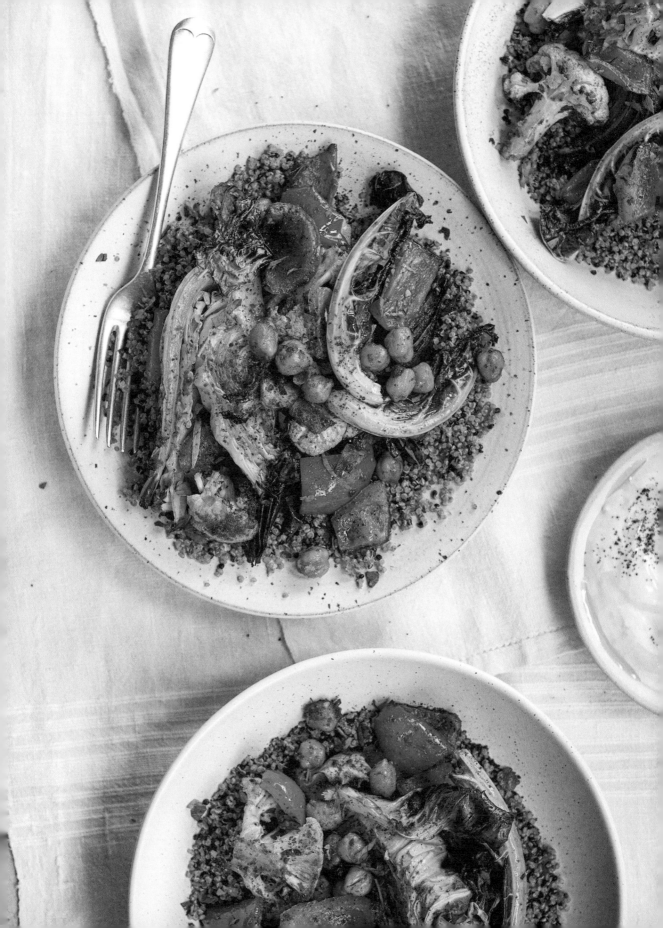

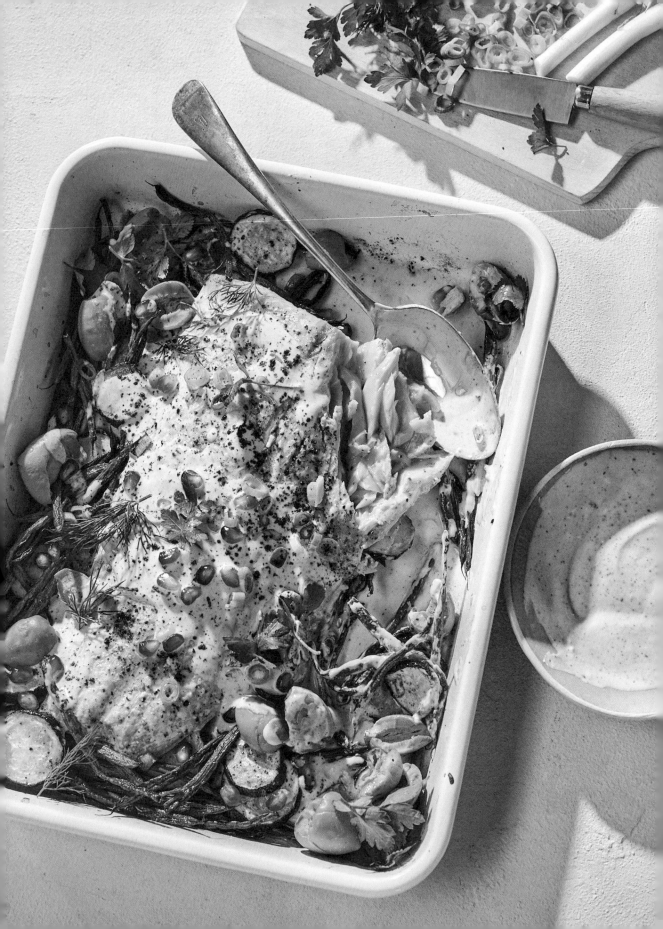

Tahini Salmon & Greens

This quick and easy dish not only looks beautiful, but is simple to make too. Perfect for a dinner party if you get a whole side of salmon—it's a showstopper.

Serves 2 | Total time: 35 minutes

7oz (200g) green beans, trimmed

1 zucchini, sliced into rounds

¼ tsp chili flakes (optional)

1 tbsp extra virgin olive oil

2 large salmon fillets

3½oz (100g) green olives

1 lemon

⅔ cup (150g) Greek yogurt

2 tbsp tahini

1 garlic clove, minced

1 tsp sumac

1 green onion, thinly sliced

large handful of pomegranate seeds

large handful of soft herbs, such as parsley, cilantro, or dill

salt and freshly ground black pepper

Preheat the oven to 400°F (200°C). Spread the green beans and zucchini slices on a large baking sheet, sprinkle with chili flakes, if using, and ½ tablespoon of the olive oil.

Roast for 20 minutes until the green beans are beginning to shrink and some corners are deeply golden.

Remove the baking sheet from the oven and nestle in the salmon fillets skin-side down with the green olives. Squeeze over the juice of half the lemon and drizzle with the remaining olive oil.

Return to the oven for 10–12 minutes until the salmon is coral and opaque.

In the meantime, whisk together the yogurt, tahini, garlic, and sumac with a generous pinch of salt and pepper. Loosen with approximately ¼ cup (60ml) cold water until you have a spoonable consistency.

Drizzle the sauce over the salmon when it comes out of the oven, and garnish with green onion, pomegranate seeds, and a scattering of herbs.

Protein | 53g/portion
Carbohydrate | 11g/portion
Fiber | 9.6g/portion

Chicken & Mushroom Pot Pie

PP
DW
LG

There's nothing better on a cozy evening than tucking into a pot pie, packed full of goodness. This pot pie uses leftover chicken, but alternatively, just buy precooked chicken breasts and shred.

Serves 4 | Total time: 1 hour

1 tbsp extra virgin olive oil

1 leek, finely sliced

1 carrot, finely diced

2 celery ribs, finely diced

1 onion, finely diced

3 garlic cloves, minced

12oz (350g) brown mushrooms

2½ tbsp Dijon mustard

1 tbsp all-purpose flour

2 cups (500ml) 2% milk

1 chicken bouillon cube or 1 tsp chicken bouillon paste

1 tbsp apple cider vinegar

1oz (25g) tarragon, tough stems removed, finely chopped

4 thyme sprigs, tough stems removed, finely chopped

1lb 2oz (500g) cooked chicken, shredded

1 x 11oz (320g) puff pastry sheet

1 egg, beaten (optional)

salt and freshly ground black pepper

TO SERVE

mixed greens

peas

mashed potato

In a 4-quart Dutch oven or a large skillet, add the oil, leek, carrot, celery, and onion. Add a big pinch of salt and cook on medium heat for 10–15 minutes, until softened and significantly reduced in volume.

Add the garlic and cook for 2 minutes until fragrant. Add the mushrooms and continue to cook for 5–10 minutes, until they are cooked through.

Dollop in the mustard and flour and stir well to coat, before gradually adding the milk, stirring well between each addition until you have a lovely thick sauce.

Dissolve the chicken bouillon cube or paste in ¼ cup (60ml) water, then add to the mixture, along with the apple cider vinegar, herbs, and chicken. Season with salt and pepper to taste.

Preheat the oven to 400°F (200°C).

Transfer the mixture to a pie or baking dish and add the puff pastry crust on top, crimping the edges with a fork. Cut a hole in the center of the pastry to allow steam to escape.

Brush with the beaten egg, if using.

Bake for 30 minutes until the crust is deeply golden and puffy.

Serve with plenty of greens and mashed potato.

Protein | 54g/portion
Carbohydrate | 47g/portion
Fiber | 4.7g/portion

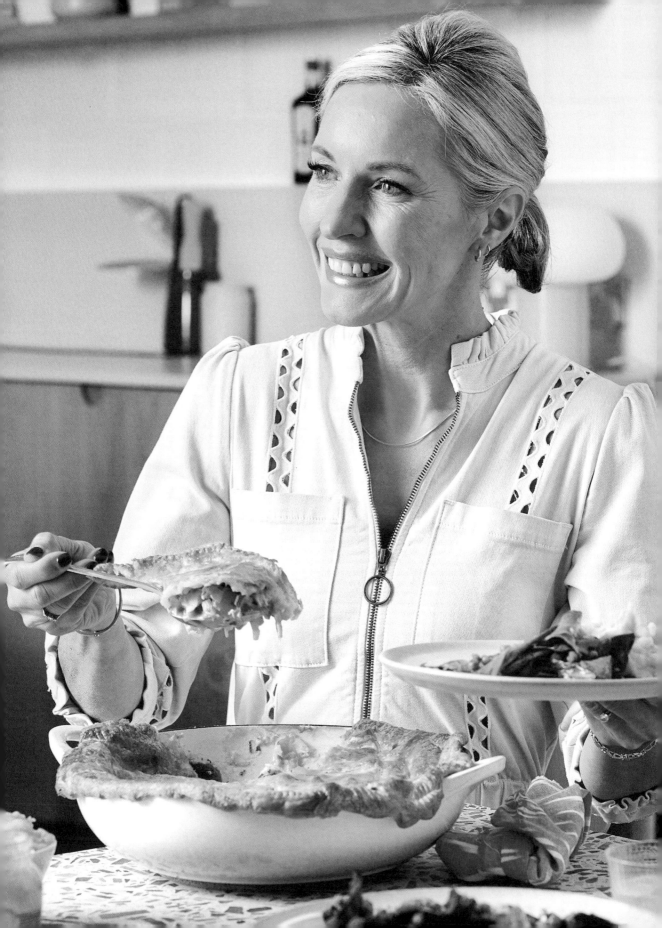

Beef & Broccoli Stir-fry

PP
DW
BS
LG

We all love stir-fries—they're so easy to whip up and a perfect way of including even more than your "five a day."

Serves 4 | **Total time: 20 minutes**

2 tbsp sesame oil

12oz (350g) steak (I like sirloin or rump), cut into strips

9oz (250g) soba noodles

1lb (450g) prepared stir-fry vegetables

2 green onions, green and white parts separated, thinly sliced

2 garlic cloves, grated

2in (5cm) piece of fresh ginger, grated

2 tbsp teriyaki marinade

2 tbsp oyster sauce

1 tbsp light soy sauce

juice of 1 lime

1 red chili, thinly sliced

sesame seeds, for sprinkling

Add the sesame oil to a wok and set on medium-high heat. Once hot, add the beef strips and cook for 8–10 minutes, until nicely seared.

Meanwhile, cook the noodles according to the package instructions and set aside until later.

Add the vegetables, white parts of the green onion, garlic, and ginger to the wok and cook for 2–3 minutes.

Add the teriyaki marinade and oyster and soy sauces and stir-fry for a final 3 minutes.

Add the cooked noodles to the wok and mix until everything comes together. Add the lime juice.

Serve garnished with the green parts of the green onion, the red chili, and sesame seeds.

Protein | 33g/portion
Carbohydrate | 55g/portion
Fiber | 8.7g/portion

Napa Cabbage with Lentils, Feta & Tahini

PP
DW
BS
WG
LG

This really is a veggie centerpiece. Charred sweetheart cabbage wedges served on a bed of lentils and brown rice with beautiful Mediterranean flavors.

Serves 4 | **Total time: 30 minutes**

1 Napa cabbage, cut into wedges

1 tbsp extra virgin olive oil

1 tsp ground cumin

1 x 9oz (250g) pouch of microwaveable brown rice

2 x 9oz (250g) pouches of cooked Puy lentils

2 green onions, finely sliced

¼ red cabbage, finely chopped

juice of 1 lemon

1¾oz (50g) tahini

2oz (60g) feta

salt

TO SERVE

1oz (30g) pistachios, coarsely chopped

pomegranate seeds

sumac

small bunch of dill or mint

Preheat the oven to 350°F (180°C).

Spread the Napa cabbage over a large baking sheet. Drizzle over the olive oil and sprinkle the cumin on top. Roast for 20–25 minutes until nicely charred.

In the meantime, heat the rice according to the package instructions. Add to a large mixing bowl along with the lentils, green onions, and red cabbage. Add half the lemon juice and season with salt.

Mix the tahini with the remaining lemon juice, then loosen with water until it is the right consistency to drizzle. Season to taste with salt.

Spoon the lentil mixture over a large platter and top with the roast Napa cabbage wedges. Drizzle over the tahini sauce and crumble over the feta.

Finish with the chopped pistachios, pomegranate seeds, sumac, and herbs.

Protein | 28g/portion
Carbohydrate | 77g/portion
Fiber | 16g/portion

Zucchini & Spicy Sausage Pasta

You can swap the sausage for chicken sausages or veggie sausages in this recipe, depending on your preference—whichever you choose, it is delicious!

Serves 4 | Total time: 30 minutes

1 tbsp olive oil

14oz (400g) low-fat pork sausages

11oz (320g) whole-grain spaghetti

3 zucchini (about 1lb 2oz/ 500g), coarsely grated

1–2 red chilies, finely chopped, to taste

3 garlic cloves, thinly sliced

zest of 1 lemon and juice of ½

2oz (60g) Parmesan cheese, grated

salt

Set a large skillet on medium-high heat and add the olive oil. Meanwhile, bring a large pan of salted water to a boil for the pasta.

Squeeze the sausage meat from the cases and add to the pan, breaking it up with a wooden spoon. Cook for 8–10 minutes until nicely browned and crispy.

Add the pasta to the boiling water and cook according to the package instructions until al dente.

In the meantime, use a slotted spoon to remove the crispy sausage meat from the pan. Set aside until later.

Add the grated zucchini to the pan and cook for 5 minutes until softened, stirring regularly. Add the chilies and garlic and cook for another 2 minutes before adding the sausage meat back into the pan. Add the lemon zest.

Drain the pasta, reserving a cup of pasta water. Add the spaghetti to the sauce along with a good splash of pasta water and toss well to coat. Add two-thirds of the Parmesan and the lemon juice, reserving the final third of Parmesan to serve.

Serve in bowls, topped with the remaining Parmesan.

Protein | 33g/portion
Carbohydrate | 61g/portion
Fiber | 13g/portion

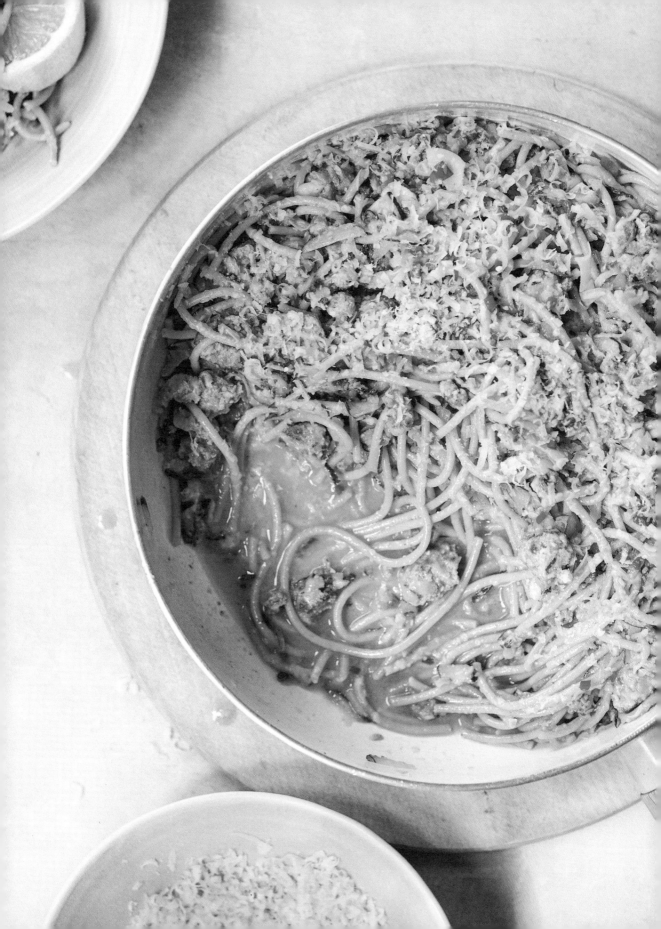

Thai Basil Shrimp Rice

PP

DW

WG

LG

This meal is delicious and really easy to put together when you need a quick fix. If you can't find Thai basil, regular basil works just fine!

Serves 2 | Total time: 15 minutes

2 tbsp oyster sauce

2 tbsp light soy sauce

1 tbsp fish sauce

juice of 1 lime

7oz (200g) bok choy or fresh spinach

½ tbsp sunflower oil

2 garlic cloves, crushed

2in (5cm) piece of fresh ginger, finely grated

1 red chili, finely chopped, plus extra to serve

1 green onion, finely sliced

5½oz (150g) raw, peeled jumbo shrimp

1 x 9oz (250g) microwaveable pouch of rice of your choice (I like brown or jasmine)

¾oz (20g) Thai basil, stems removed

lime wedges to serve (optional)

To start, mix together the oyster sauce, soy sauce, fish sauce, and lime juice. Set aside.

Finely slice the stalks of the bok choy and keep the leaves whole. Set aside.

Add the oil to a large wok or skillet, then fry the bok choy stalks, garlic, ginger, chili, and green onion on high heat for 1 minute until fragrant.

Add the shrimp and bok choy leaves and stir-fry for 2–3 minutes, until the shrimp is pink and cooked through.

Microwave the rice according to the package instructions.

Add the sauce and most of the Thai basil leaves to the shrimp, warm through, and wilt. Remove from the heat and serve with the rice and an additional sprinkle of Thai basil leaves, chopped chili, and lime wedges, if using.

Protein | 27g/portion
Carbohydrate | 99g/portion
Fiber | 6.8g/portion

Tuna Puttanesca Pasta

PP
DW
BS
LG

Puttanesca is one of my ultimate pasta dishes, and with tuna and a pea-based pasta, it really packs in the protein too.

Serves 2 | Total time: 20 minutes

1 tbsp olive oil

2 garlic cloves, sliced

2 anchovy fillets

1 x 14oz (400g) can of diced tomatoes

1 tbsp capers

1¼oz (40g) Kalamata olives, pitted

7oz (200g) gluten-free pasta (I use pea pasta)

2 x 5oz (145g) cans of tuna in water

juice of 1 lemon, plus extra (optional) to serve

3½oz (100g) baby spinach

½oz (15g) basil, leaves picked and torn

2 tbsp grated Parmesan cheese

salt and freshly ground black pepper

Add the olive oil to a large skillet and cook the garlic and anchovies on medium heat for 2 minutes until fragrant, mashing down the anchovies with the back of your wooden spoon until they melt into the oil.

Add the tomatoes and rinse out the can with 1 cup (200ml) water and allow to cook until reduced, about 10 minutes. Add the capers and tear in the olives.

Bring a large pan of salted water to a boil and cook the pasta according to the package instructions.

While the pasta is cooking, add the tuna to the tomato mixture, season with the lemon juice, and add the spinach. Once the spinach has wilted, tear in the basil and season to taste with salt and pepper. Using a slotted spoon, add the pasta straight from the water into the sauce and toss well to combine, using a few cups of pasta water if necessary to loosen and make the dish nice and glossy.

Serve with a sprinkling of the Parmesan and extra lemon juice, if you like.

Protein | 45g/portion
Carbohydrate | 35g/portion
Fiber | 9.8g/portion

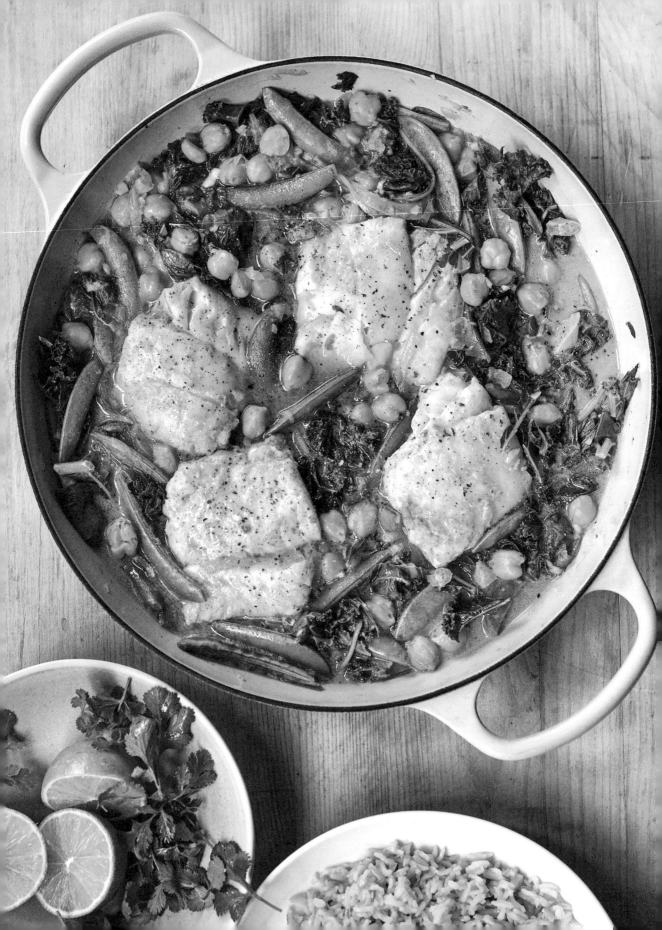

Fragrant Coconut Curry with Cod

This delicately spiced curry is my ultimate midweek dinner—not too hot, but instead zesty, fragrant, and aromatic. Use any firm white fish that you like here, or it would be lovely with salmon too.

Serves 4 | Total time: 35 minutes

1 tbsp coconut oil

1 onion, thinly sliced

1¾oz (50g) fresh ginger, finely grated

4 garlic cloves, minced

1 green chili, finely chopped

1 tbsp ground turmeric

1 tbsp medium curry powder

1¾ cups (400ml) coconut milk

¾ cup (200ml) vegetable stock

1 x 14.5oz (425g) can of chickpeas, drained and rinsed

4 skinless cod fillets

7oz (200g) sugar snap peas

3½oz (100g) kale, tough stems removed and coarsely chopped

3½oz (100g) fresh spinach

juice of 2 limes

salt

TO SERVE

brown rice

½oz (15g) cilantro, coarsely chopped

Heat the coconut oil in a large, high-sided skillet and add the onion and a pinch of salt. Cook on medium heat for 10–15 minutes until softened.

Add the ginger, garlic, and chili and cook for 2 minutes, then add the turmeric and curry powder and cook for another minute.

Pour in the coconut milk and vegetable stock and bubble for 5 minutes.

Add the chickpeas and nestle in the cod fillets. Reduce the heat to simmer and cook for 6 minutes.

Add the sugar snap peas, kale, and spinach to the pan and slowly incorporate into the sauce. Cook for a final 3–4 minutes until wilted and the fish is flaking and fully cooked. Squeeze in the lime juice.

Serve the curry with brown rice and cilantro.

Protein | 35g/portion
Carbohydrate | 30g/portion
Fiber | 12g/portion

Socca Pizza

PP

DW

BS

In areas of Southern France and Northern Italy they make the most delicious sandwiches using socca—a chickpea flour pancake. Here, I've topped the socca like a pizza for a great high-protein alternative to traditional dough. It's very quick to whip up and gluten-free to boot!

Serves 4 | Total time: 40 minutes

2½ cups (320g) chickpea (gram) flour

1 tsp fine salt

2 tbsp olive oil

1 x 14oz (411g) can of diced tomatoes

1 tsp dried oregano

1 garlic clove, grated

9oz (250g) ricotta

9½oz (280g) sun-dried tomatoes, drained and patted dry of excess oil

handful of pitted green olives, halved

1¼oz (40g) arugula

balsamic glaze or pesto of your choice, to serve (optional)

flaky sea salt

Add the flour to a mixing bowl with the fine salt, then pour in 2 cups (500ml) of water. Stir to combine and make a batter.

Set a medium-sized skillet on medium-high heat and add ½ tablespoon of olive oil. Once hot, add a quarter of the batter to the pan and cook for 3–4 minutes, then use a spatula to flip over and cook for another 1–2 minutes. Meanwhile, preheat the broiler to high.

In a medium-sized bowl, combine the tomatoes with the dried oregano, garlic, and a generous pinch of salt. Spoon this over the socca base, then top with a quarter of the ricotta. Scatter over a quarter of the sun-dried tomatoes and olives.

Slide the skillet under the broiler and cook for 2 minutes.

Remove from the broiler and top with some arugula. Finish with a drizzle of balsamic glaze or pesto if you like. Repeat with the remaining batter and toppings, adding ½ tablespoon of oil to the pan for cooking each pancake.

Protein | 43g/portion
Carbohydrate | 68g/portion
Fiber | 17g/portion

Sheetpan Sausage & Kraut

These flavors taste like fall on a plate. Perfect for getting cozy, while taking care of your belly, with some delivious fermented food, veggies, and pulses.

Serves 4 | Total time: 40 minutes

8 pork sausages

9oz (250g) cherry tomatoes

7oz (200g) Brussels sprouts, halved

1 x 14.5oz (425g) can of butter beans, drained

1 red onion, cut into wedges

2 sprigs of rosemary

3 tbsp extra virgin olive oil

7oz (200g) sauerkraut

1 tbsp whole-grain mustard

1 tbsp apple cider vinegar

1 tsp maple syrup

Preheat the oven to 375°F (190°C).

Arrange the sausages, cherry tomatoes, Brussels sprouts, butter beans, and red onion on a large baking sheet. Sprinkle with the leaves from the rosemary sprigs and drizzle with 1 tablespoon of the olive oil.

Bake for 25–30 minutes until golden.

In the meantime, add the sauerkraut to a small bowl and mix with the mustard, apple cider vinegar, remaining olive oil, and the maple syrup.

Serve with the sheetpan sausage and enjoy.

Protein | 25g/portion
Carbohydrate | 36g/portion
Fiber | 15g/portion

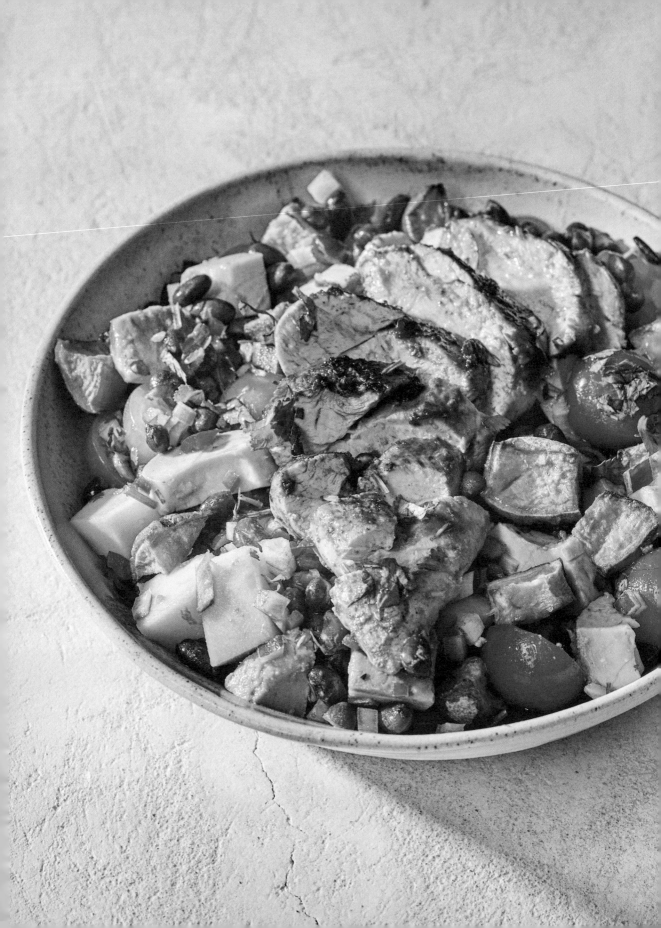

Chipotle Chicken Bowl

This dense bean salad, packed with flavor and protein, will keep you full and satisfied for a long time.

Serves 2 | Total time: 35 minutes

1 sweet potato, cubed

½ tbsp olive oil

1 tsp ground cumin

½ red onion, finely diced

zest and juice of 2 limes

2 skinless chicken breasts

1 tbsp adobo sauce

½ tbsp olive oil

1 x 15oz (425g) can of black beans, drained and rinsed

9oz (250g) mango, diced

1 avocado, diced or sliced

7oz (200g) cherry tomatoes, halved

large handful of cilantro, finely chopped

½ red chili, finely chopped (optional)

salt and freshly ground black pepper

Toss the sweet potato cubes with the olive oil and cumin. Air-fry at 350°F (180°C) for 12–15 minutes, or bake in the oven at 350°F (180°C) for 15–20 minutes until tender and golden.

In the meantime, add the red onion to a large bowl with the zest and juice of both limes. Set aside to pickle slightly.

Season the chicken breasts and rub the adobo sauce over them, then heat the remaining olive oil in a skillet and cook the chicken for 2–3 minutes on each side, until cooked through and slightly charred on the outside. Set aside to rest.

Add the black beans, mango, avocado, tomatoes, and sweet potato to the large bowl with the onion. Toss everything to combine.

Divide the salad between bowls and top each one with a sliced chicken breast. Garnish with the cilantro and chili, if you like. Enjoy.

Protein | 52g/portion
Carbohydrate | 75g/portion
Fiber | 24g/portion

Tofu & Pineapple Stir-fry

Sweet and tangy with incredible textures, this is a speedy vegan delight.

PP
DW
BS
LG

Serves 2 | Total time: 20 minutes

2 tbsp sesame oil

10oz (300g) extra-firm tofu, patted dry and cubed

1 lemongrass, tough stem removed and thinly sliced

2 garlic cloves, finely chopped

1 red chili, finely chopped

2 x 8oz (220g) packages of stir-fry vegetables

10oz (300g) fresh pineapple, cubed

2 tbsp light soy sauce

2 tbsp reduced-sugar sweet chili sauce

2 nests instant rice noodles

juice of 1 lime

small handful of cilantro, coarsely chopped

1 lime, cut into wedges (optional)

½ red chili, finely chopped (optional)

Add 1 tablespoon of the sesame oil to a wok and set on medium-high heat. Once hot, add the tofu and cook for 2–3 minutes on each side until golden. Remove and set aside until later.

Add the remaining sesame oil to the wok, then add the lemongrass, garlic, and chili. Cook for 2 minutes.

Add the vegetables and pineapple to the wok, along with the soy sauce and sweet chili sauce. Cook for 5 minutes.

Meanwhile, cook the noodles according to the package instructions.

Add the cooked noodles to the wok and stir to combine. Add the lime juice.

Finally, divide the noodles between two serving bowls, top with the tofu, and garnish with the chopped cilantro. Serve with lime wedges and finely chopped red chili, if you'd like.

Protein | 38g/portion
Carbohydrate | 75g/portion
Fiber | 13g/portion

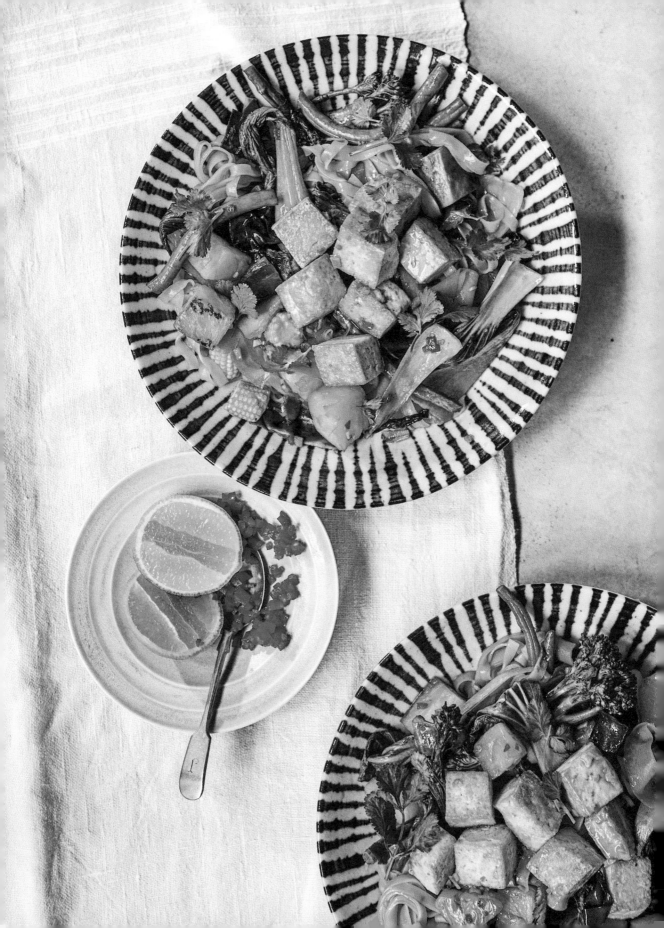

Eggplant Satay Curry

PP
DW
BS
WG
LG

1 tbsp coconut oil

14oz (400g) baby eggplant, left whole with stalk intact

1¾ cups (400ml) coconut milk

10oz (300g) silken tofu

⅓ cup (80g) peanut butter

2 tbsp vegan fish sauce

1 tbsp light soy sauce

juice of 2 limes

4 garlic cloves, grated

2in (5cm) piece of fresh ginger, finely grated

1 red chili, finely chopped

4 fresh makrut lime leaves, shredded

¾ cup (200ml) vegetable stock

7oz (200g) green beans, trimmed and cut in half

6oz (175g) baby corn, halved lengthwise

2 bok choy, quartered

TO SERVE

brown rice

1¾oz (50g) salted roasted peanuts, coarsely chopped

small bunch of cilantro, coarsely chopped

This coconut and peanut curry is so creamy and delicious, and I've found a way of sneaking in more protein by blending silken tofu into the sauce. You can't taste it, it just adds a richness and depth to the dish.

Serves 4 | Total time: 40 minutes

Heat the coconut oil in a large pan on medium-high heat. Once hot, add the baby eggplants and cook for 8–10 minutes, until nicely browned on all sides.

Meanwhile, make the satay sauce. Combine the coconut milk, tofu, peanut butter, vegan fish sauce, soy sauce, and lime juice in a blender and pulse to combine.

Add the garlic, ginger, red chili, and lime leaves to the eggplant and cook for 2 minutes.

Pour in the satay sauce along with the vegetable stock and bring to a gentle simmer for 25 minutes, until the eggplants are almost cooked through.

At this stage, add the green beans, baby corn, and bok choy and cook for a final 3–4 minutes.

Serve the curry with brown rice and topped with the peanuts and chopped cilantro.

Protein | 18g/portion
Carbohydrate | 18g/portion
Fiber | 8.9g/portion

Sheetpan Chicken & Chorizo

These Spanish-inspired flavors are totally heavenly for a sheetpan supper; I love the richness from the rye bread in the crumb coating and Manchego is simply a wonderful cheese to sprinkle on any dish. Swap the zucchini and asparagus for any other green veggies when they're out of season.

Serves 4 | Total time: 45 minutes

1lb 12oz (800g) baby potatoes, halved

1 tbsp extra virgin olive oil

1 slice of rye bread, torn into chunks

2½oz (75g) chorizo sausage, coarsely chopped

1 garlic clove

handful of flat-leaf parsley, coarsely chopped, a few leaves reserved for garnish

4 skinless chicken breasts

1 zucchini, sliced into rounds

5½oz (150g) asparagus spears

2 roasted red bell peppers, thinly sliced

½oz (15g) Manchego cheese, grated

salt and freshly ground black pepper

Preheat the oven to 375°F (190°C).

Toss the baby potatoes in the olive oil on a large flat baking sheet and roast for 25 minutes.

In the meantime, add the rye bread, chorizo, garlic, and parsley to a blender or food processor and whiz together until you have a fragrant bread-crumb mixture.

After 25 minutes, add the chicken, zucchini, and asparagus to the baking sheet. Season well. Sprinkle the chorizo crumb onto the chicken breasts and return the baking sheet to the oven for another 15–20 minutes, until the chicken is cooked through.

When you pull the baking sheet out of the oven, sprinkle over the roasted bell peppers, grated Manchego, and reserved parsley.

Protein | 43g/portion
Carbohydrate | 41g/portion
Fiber | 5.6g/portion

Beef & Lentil Lasagne

1 tbsp extra virgin olive oil

2 large carrots, finely chopped

2 celery ribs, finely chopped

1 onion, finely chopped

½ fennel bulb, finely chopped

3½oz (100g) shiitake mushrooms, finely chopped

a few sprigs of thyme, leaves picked and finely chopped

a few sprigs of rosemary, leaves picked and finely chopped

a few sprigs of oregano, leaves picked and finely chopped

4 garlic cloves, finely grated or crushed

1lb 2oz (500g) lean (5%) ground beef

¾ cup (200g) canned brown or green lentils

2 x 14oz (411g) cans of diced tomatoes

2 tbsp red wine vinegar

1 tbsp brewer's yeast

1 beef bouillon cube

10oz (300g) dried whole-wheat ready-to-bake lasagne sheets

salt and freshly ground black pepper

2oz (60g) Parmesan cheese, finely grated, plus extra to serve

FOR THE WHITE SAUCE

1lb 2oz (500g) ricotta cheese

⅔ cup (150ml) whole milk

1 egg

1½ tsp Dijon mustard

I love to increase the amount of vegetables in my favorite meals, and making a big batch of ragù that's half veg and half meat is such an easy way to get there. You can also skip the lasagne part and use this as a lovely Bolognese with rice, pasta, or on a baked sweet potato.

Serves 6–8 | Total time: 1¾ hours

Add the oil to a large deep saucepan and add the carrots, celery, onion, fennel, and mushrooms. Cook on medium heat for 10–15 minutes, until softened and reduced in volume, then add the herbs and garlic and cook for another 2 minutes until fragrant.

Add the ground beef and break it up with the back of your spoon until it has a crumbly texture, then follow with the lentils. Add the canned tomatoes and a can full of water.

Add the vinegar, brewer's yeast, and bouillon cube and season with a pinch of salt and pepper. Cover and leave to simmer for at least 45 minutes, or up to 2 hours, until tender.

In the meantime, mix together the ricotta, milk, egg, mustard, and Parmesan and season. Set aside.

Preheat the oven to 350°F (180°C).

To assemble the lasagne, add a thin layer of the meat sauce to the bottom of a large deep baking pan, followed by a layer of lasagne sheets (you may have to break some to make them fit). Continue this layering process until the lasagne is about ⅜in (1.5cm) from the top. Ending with a layer of pasta sheets, spoon over all of the white sauce and the Parmesan, then return to the oven for 40 minutes. Slice and enjoy.

Protein | 53g/portion
Carbohydrate | 41g/portion
Fiber | 8.6g/portion

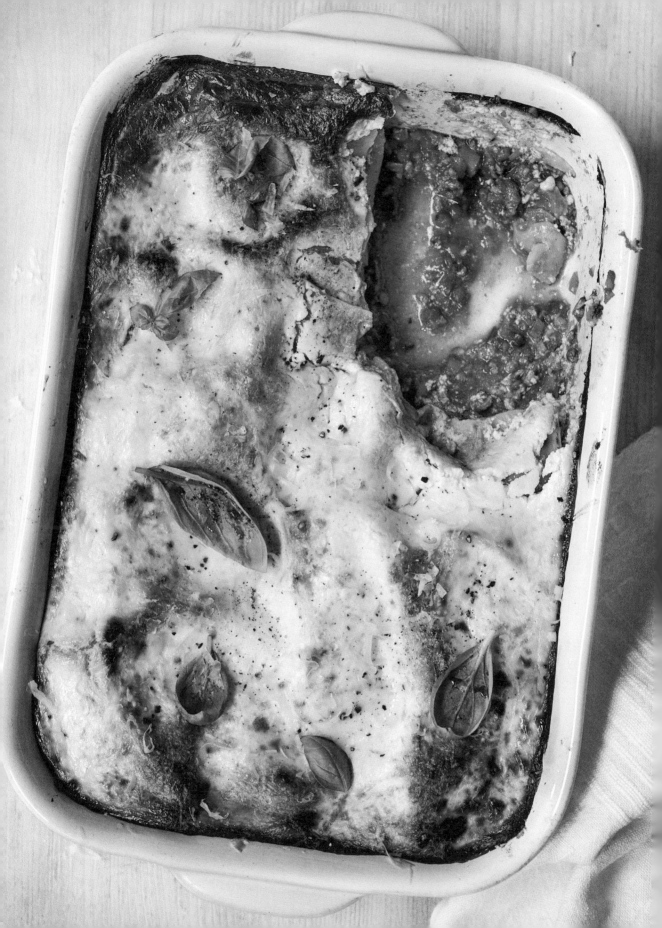

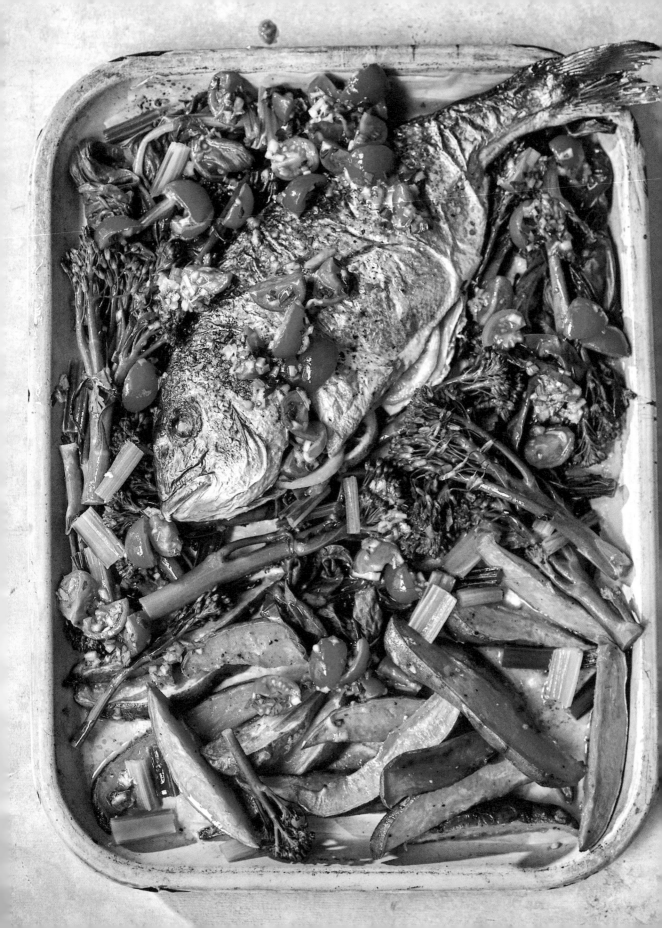

Roasted Sea Bream with Greens & Tomato Salsa Verde

PP DW BS LG

There's nothing I love more than tucking into a whole fish at supper. This zingy and fresh tomato-packed salsa verde is a really great relish that I put on lots of my meals, so make a double batch if you like!

Serves 2 | Total time: 40 minutes

2 sweet potatoes, cut into wedges

1½ tbsp extra virgin olive oil

7oz (200g) Swiss chard or kale, stems coarsely chopped and leaves kept whole

7oz (200g) broccolini

1 large or 2 smaller sea bream or sea bass, gutted

½ lemon, sliced

salt and freshly ground black pepper

FOR THE TOMATO SALSA VERDE

1 shallot, finely diced

3 tbsp red wine vinegar

1 tsp Dijon mustard

1 tbsp extra virgin olive oil

1 tsp maple syrup

7oz (200g) cherry tomatoes, quartered

large handful of flat-leaf parsley, finely chopped

Preheat the oven to 350°F (180°C).

In a large roasting pan, toss the sweet potato wedges in ½ tablespoon of the olive oil and season with salt and pepper. Roast for 15 minutes.

In the meantime, make the tomato salsa verde by adding the shallot and red wine vinegar to a small bowl and set aside.

After 15 minutes, add the Swiss chard and broccolini to the pan. Fill the cavity of the fish with the lemon slices and nestle the fish on top of the vegetables. Season again with salt and pepper and drizzle with the remaining tablespoon of olive oil. Cook for 12–15 minutes, until the fish flesh is white and flaking away from the bone.

While the fish is cooking, add the mustard, oil, maple syrup, cherry tomatoes, and parsley to the bowl of shallot and mix well to combine.

Remove from the oven. Enjoy the fish with the tomato salsa verde.

Protein | 31g/portion
Carbohydrate | 60g/portion
Fiber | 15g/portion

Smoothies, 2 Ways

*This vivid purple drink is one of my favorite smoothies—earthy,
sweet, and invigorating. My other go-to drink is a green smoothie.
I've got a powerful blender so I like to add the kiwis with the skin for
the extra fiber, but if you find the texture off-putting, just peel them!*

Makes 1 large smoothie (each flavor) | Total time: 5 minutes

Beet & Blackberry

5½oz (150g) blackberries

9oz (250g) cooked beets

2 tbsp milled flaxseeds

2in (5cm) piece of fresh ginger

2 dried dates, pitted

1 cup (250ml) soy milk

Put all the ingredients into a blender and
pulse until smooth.

Pour into a glass and enjoy.

PP

DW

BS

O3

Protein | 14g/portion
Carbohydrate | 46g/portion
Fiber | 19g/portion

Green

1 avocado

2 kiwis

juice of 1 lemon

2in (5cm) of fresh ginger

*1 cup (250ml) almond milk or
cashew milk*

1¼oz (40g) spinach

*1 tbsp protein powder of your
choice (except chocolate)*

Put all the ingredients into a blender and pulse
until smooth. Loosen, if you need to, with up to
½ cup (100ml) of water.

Pour into a glass and enjoy.

PP

DW

BS

LG

Protein | 31g/portion
Carbohydrate | 16g/portion
Fiber | 8.6g/portion

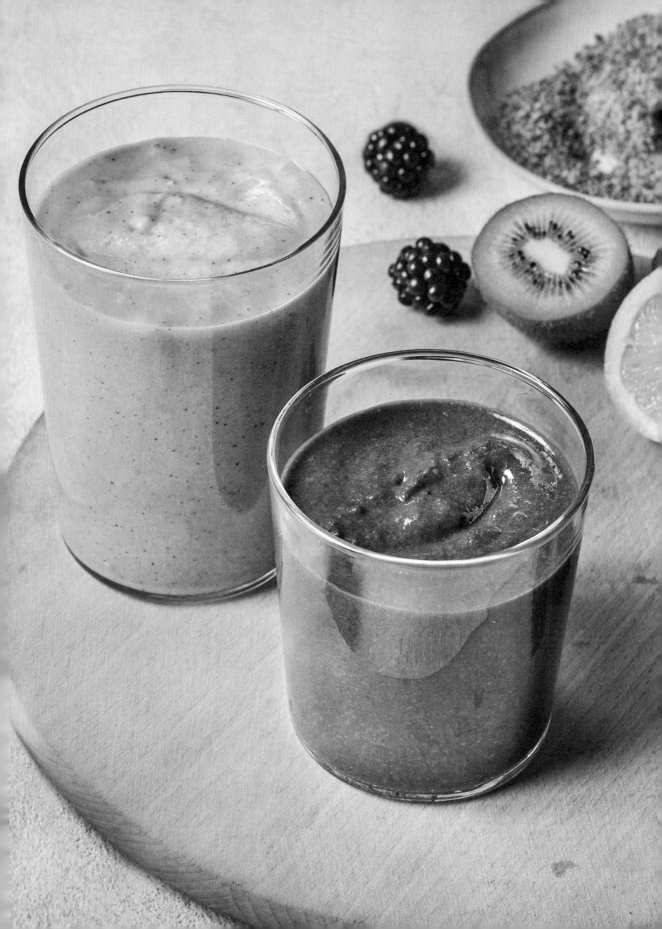

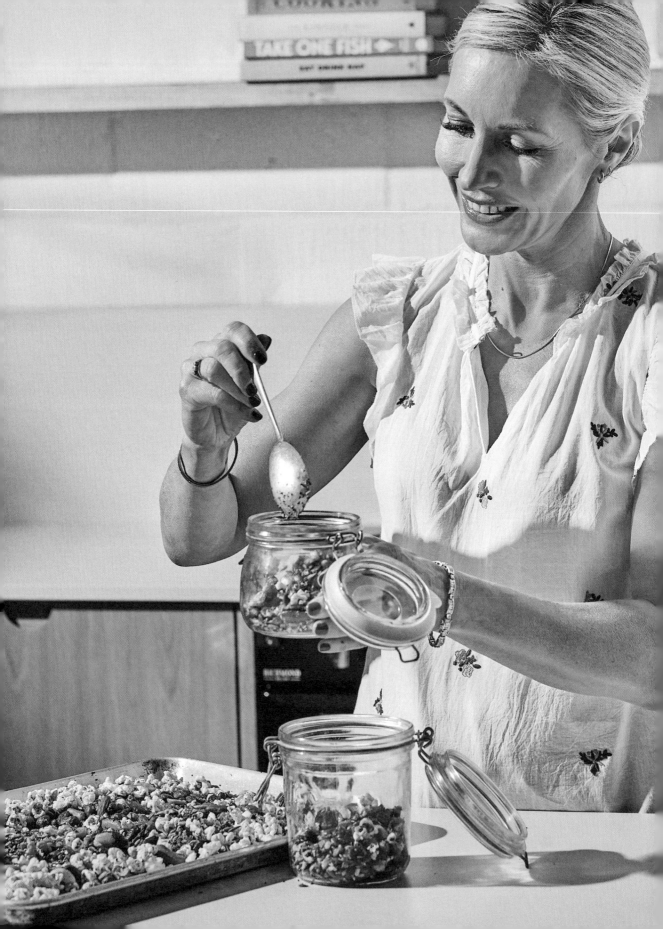

Protein Trail Mix

This flavor-packed trail mix is the perfect batch snack, as nutritional yeast is packed with vitamins, minerals, and protein and gives this mix a lovely flavor. Swap the other ingredients for anything you have in the cupboard—crackers, crispy chickpeas, even dried fruit.

Makes 8 servings | Total time: 30 minutes

1oz (30g) salted popped popcorn

2¼ cups (300g) mixed nuts (I used almonds, cashews, and walnuts)

5 tbsp mixed seeds or seed topper (I used sunflower, pumpkin, sesame, and linseed)

2 tbsp chia seeds

3 tbsp nutritional yeast

1 tsp garlic powder

¼ tsp salt

1½ tbsp extra virgin olive oil

Preheat the oven to 350°F (180°C).

Pour all the ingredients into a large bowl and mix well to coat in the olive oil. Spread out on a large baking sheet.

Roast for 25 minutes, until lightly golden and fragrant. Allow to cool fully, then store in an airtight container for up to 2 weeks.

Protein | 19g/portion
Carbohydrate | 10g/portion
Fiber | 8.6g/portion

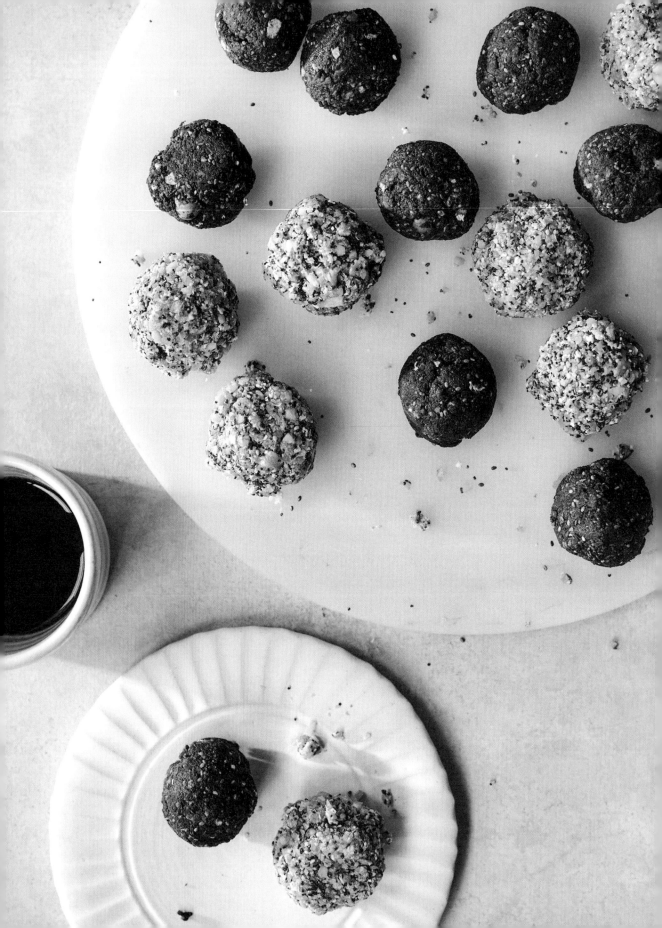

Energy Bites, 2 Ways

Energy bites are a great thing to have in your back pocket. They're packed with goodness and perfect for filling in those gaps between mealtimes.

Makes 12 (each flavor) | **Total time: 10 minutes (each)**

Mocha Hazelnut

5½oz (150g) pitted Medjool dates

1 cup (100g) rolled oats

2 tbsp chia seeds

2 tbsp cocoa powder

3½oz (100g) hazelnuts

1 tbsp instant coffee powder

Add all the ingredients to a blender and pulse to combine. If your dates aren't very sticky, you may need a few tablespoons of water to allow the mixture to come together. Start with 2 tablespoons and go from there—you want the mixture to feel like just-damp sand that holds together when squeezed.

Roll into 12 balls and refrigerate for up to a week.

PP
DW
BS
WG
O3

Protein | 3.1g/ball
Carbohydrate | 15g/ball
Fiber | 2.8g/ball

Lemon & Poppy Seed

1 cup (100g) rolled oats

5½oz (150g) dried apricots

2 tbsp chia seeds

2 tbsp poppy seeds

zest and juice of 2 small lemons

3½oz (100g) cashews

Add all the ingredients to a blender and pulse to combine. If your apricots aren't very sticky, you may need a few tablespoons of water to allow the mixture to come together. Start with ½ tablespoon and go from there—you want the mixture to feel like just-damp sand that holds together when squeezed.

Roll into 12 balls and refrigerate for up to a week.

PP
DW
BS
WG
O3

Protein | 3.9g/ball
Carbohydrate | 13g/ball
Fiber | 2.9g/ball

My Tracker Bars

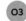

Making your own protein and energy bars is a real game-changer and just so much better for you than the store-bought alternatives. I love keeping these in the freezer to grab and go—or keep in the fridge if you like a slightly softer texture.

Makes 14 | Total time: 1 hour plus freezing

1oz (25g) coconut oil

½ cup (150g) smooth peanut butter

6oz (170g) honey

1 cup (100g) puffed whole-grain rice

3½oz (100g) unsalted peanuts

1oz (25g) sunflower seeds

1oz (25g) pumpkin seeds

¾oz (20g) chia seeds

¾oz (20g) flaxseeds

pinch of salt

TO COAT (optional)

2oz (60g) 70% dark chocolate

1 tbsp coconut oil

Line an 8in (20cm) square baking pan with parchment paper.

In a small saucepan, melt together the coconut oil, peanut butter, and honey. Alternatively, you can do this in a heatproof bowl in the microwave in 20-second bursts, stirring between each one.

Add all the remaining ingredients to a large bowl and pour over the melted peanut butter mixture and stir well to combine.

Press the mixture into the lined pan and refrigerate for 30 minutes–2 hours, until firm to the touch and cool.

If coating, add the chocolate and coconut oil to a small heatproof bowl and melt together in the microwave in 20-second bursts, stirring between each one.

Turn the seedy mixture onto a cutting board and slice into 14 bars. Dip the base of each bar into the chocolate, then place them on a large baking sheet lined with parchment paper spaced well apart. Freeze until set. You can then transfer them into sandwich bags and they will keep for up to 2 months in the freezer or for 2 weeks in the fridge.

Protein | 6.4g/portion
Carbohydrate | 19g/portion
Fiber | 3.2g/portion

Protein-packed Guacamole

I was so happy to discover that you can seamlessly blend silken tofu into guacamole—it is totally undetectable, and TOTALLY delectable—an amazing way to pump up the nutritional value of this party staple.

Serves 4 | Total time: 15 minutes

5½oz (150g) silken tofu, drained

2 avocados

juice of 1–2 limes, to taste

1 small red onion, very finely diced

1¾oz (50g) cherry tomatoes, quartered

1 red chili, finely diced

small bunch of cilantro, finely chopped, plus a few leaves to garnish

flaky sea salt

tortilla chips, to serve

Add the tofu, half an avocado, and the juice of half a lime to a high-speed blender and blend until smooth. Transfer to a bowl.

Coarsely mash the remaining avocado, keeping it quite chunky. Add this to the tofu and avocado mixture along with most of the red onion and cherry tomatoes, the red chili, and the finely chopped cilantro.

Squeeze in more lime juice and season with salt, tasting and adding more of both as necessary.

Serve with the reserved red onion, tomatoes, and chopped cilantro scattered on top, with tortilla chips for scooping up the guacamole.

Protein | 3.6g/portion
Carbohydrate | 4.9g/portion
Fiber | 2.7g/portion

Beet Hummus Mezze Plate

PP

DW

BS

This beautiful mezze plate is one to definitely include in this book!
Use whatever veggies you love and fill your plate with color. This
recipe makes more than one serving of hummus, so store half of it in
a jar and consider it prepped to enjoy throughout the week. You can
include some whole-grain carb dipping choices to add more fiber and
balance, e.g., whole-grain bread sticks, seeded rye crackers, or
oatcakes. Baby corn is a good addition to the veggie selection.

Serves 2 | Total time: 15 minutes

FOR THE HUMMUS

7oz (200g) store-bought
hummus (see Tip)

9oz (250g) cooked beets

juice of ½ lemon

2½oz (75g) sunflower seeds

1 tsp za'atar or dukkah

1 tsp extra virgin olive oil

salt and freshly ground
black pepper

FOR THE MEZZE PLATE
CHOOSE FROM:

baby cucumbers, baby corn,
carrots, bell peppers, sugar
snap peas, endive, radishes,
cherry tomatoes, celery ribs,
olives, falafel

Add the hummus, beets, lemon juice, and sunflower seeds,
reserving a few to garnish, to a high-powered blender and pulse
together until the mixture is vibrantly pink. Season to taste, then
transfer to a small bowl.

Sprinkle with za'atar or dukkah, the remaining sunflower seeds, and
drizzle over the olive oil.

Cut and prep your veggies of choice, arrange them beautifully on a
platter, and get dipping!

Hot tip

Where possible, buy low-fat
hummus, as it contains all the
good stuff, with a little less
oil. Better still, make it yourself
at home!

Protein | 18g/portion
Carbohydrate | 29g/portion
Fiber | 11g/portion

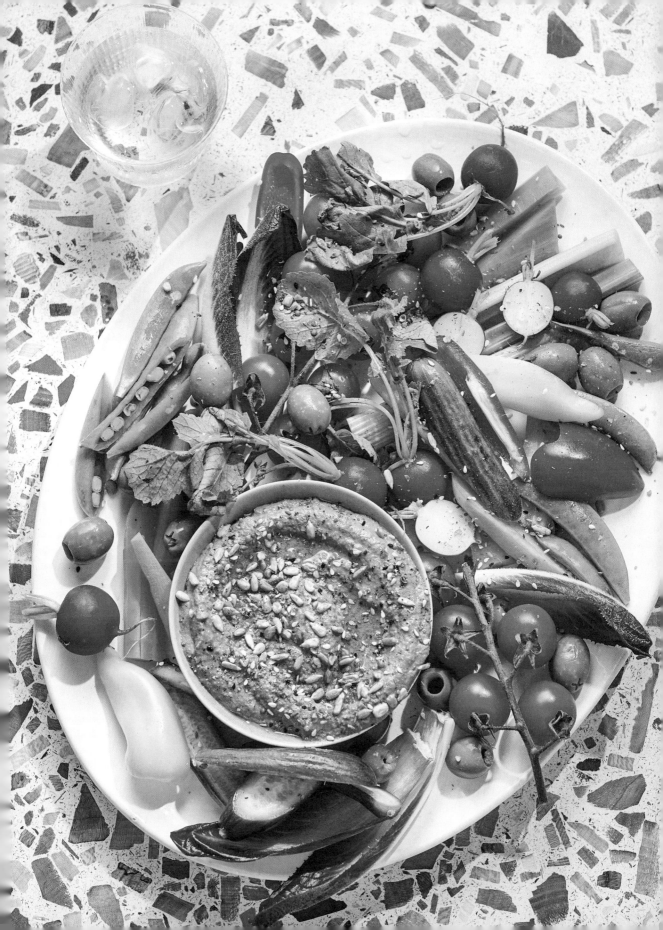

Whipped Feta & Smoked Salmon

PP
BS
O3

As soon as I discovered you could whip cottage cheese, I was hooked—it's so creamy. Here it's whipped with feta and lots of lemon zest for a delicious spread that you can keep in the fridge and spread on veggies, crackers, or toast for a quick high-protein snack. For this, I've paired it with smoked salmon and cucumber.

Makes 8 crackers | **Total time: 15 minutes**

FOR THE WHIPPED FETA

9oz (250g) fat-free cottage cheese

2½oz (75g) feta

zest of 1 lemon, lemon sliced for serving

freshly ground black pepper

FOR THE CRACKERS

8 multi-grain crispbread crackers

¾oz (20g) smoked salmon per cracker

½ cucumber, sliced very thinly

a few sprigs of dill or a pinch of finely chopped chives

a drizzle of extra virgin olive oil

Add the cottage cheese, feta, and lemon zest to a blender and whiz until smooth.

To assemble your snack, spread 2 tablespoons of the whipped feta on a multi-grain crispbread cracker and top with smoked salmon and a few cucumber slices and dill leaves. Serve with a lemon wedge for squeezing on top and a grind of black pepper. Leftover whipped feta will keep in an airtight container in the fridge for up to a week.

Protein	10g/portion
Carbohydrate	6.8g/portion
Fiber	0.5g/portion

Hot tip

If you're not a fan of cottage cheese, use Greek yogurt instead, or do half and half!

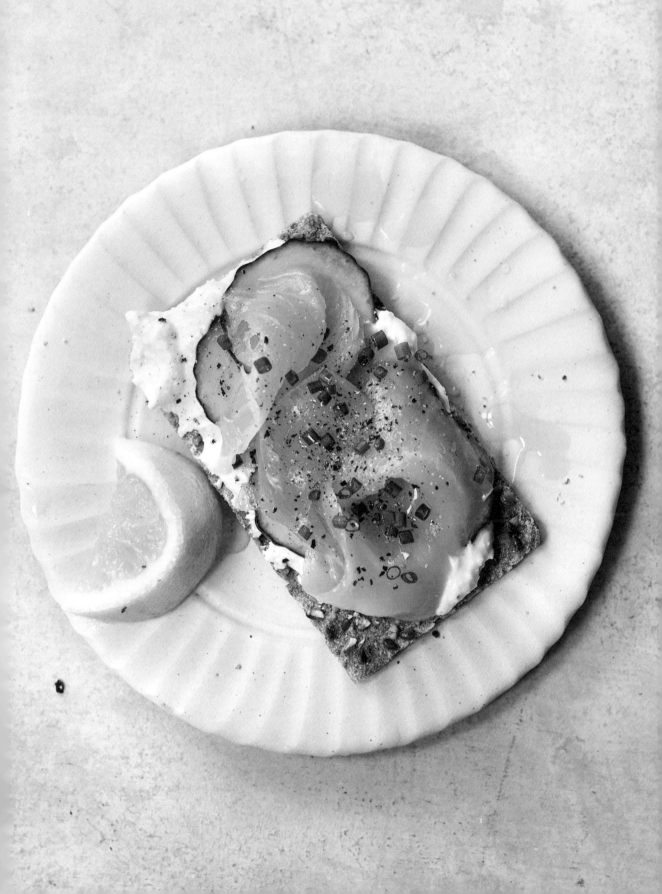

Canned Fish Temaki

PP
DW
BS
O3

Like sushi, but it's ten times easier. Open a can of fish from the cupboard, mix it, and roll it up in a half sheet of nori.

Makes 6 rolls | Total time: 5 minutes

1 x 5oz (145g) can of salmon or tuna, drained

2 tbsp Greek yogurt

1 tbsp sriracha

6 half-cut nori sheets

⅛ cucumber, sliced into thin batons

1 green onion, shredded

1 tbsp sesame seeds

Mix the drained fish with the yogurt and sriracha to combine.

Place a few tablespoons of the fish mixture in the left-hand center of a nori sheet, shiny-side down. Top with a few batons of cucumber and some green onion slices.

Fold the bottom left corner up and over the filling to roll it into a cone shape. Use a slightly damp finger to seal the roll closed.

Sprinkle with sesame seeds and enjoy. Repeat with the remaining filling and nori sheets.

Protein | 7.7g/roll
Carbohydrate | 1.3g/roll
Fiber | 1.4g/roll

Antipasto Roll-ups

*These little roll-ups are the perfect thing to rustle up when you're
standing in front of the fridge trying to make a healthy choice.
Quick, easy, heaven.*

Makes 4 roll-ups | Total time: 5 minutes

2 tsp Dijon mustard

*4 Baby Gem or butter lettuce
leaves*

2 slices of cheese of your choice

4 slices of ham

8 pitted green olives

4 large basil leaves

It's as simple as spreading a little bit of mustard onto the lettuce
leaf, then topping with half a slice of cheese, a slice of ham, a few
torn olives, and a basil leaf. Roll up to enjoy instantly.

Protein | 8.8g/roll-up
Carbohydrate | 4.6g/roll-up
Fiber | 5.4g/roll-up

Protein Raspberry Fruit Dip

Sometimes, you just don't feel like a savory dip. Here's a great fruit alternative.

Serves 2 | **Total time: 10 minutes**

¾ cup (200g) Greek yogurt

3½oz (100g) raspberries

1 scoop of your favorite protein powder

1 tsp ground cardamom

3 tbsp tahini

14oz (400g) fruit of your choice (I like melon, pineapple, berries, and grapes)

Add the yogurt, raspberries, protein powder, cardamom, and tahini to a blender and pulse until combined and smooth. Transfer to a bowl.

Cut your favorite fruit into batons and dip away!

Protein | 28g/portion
Carbohydrate | 27g/portion
Fiber | 7.8g/portion

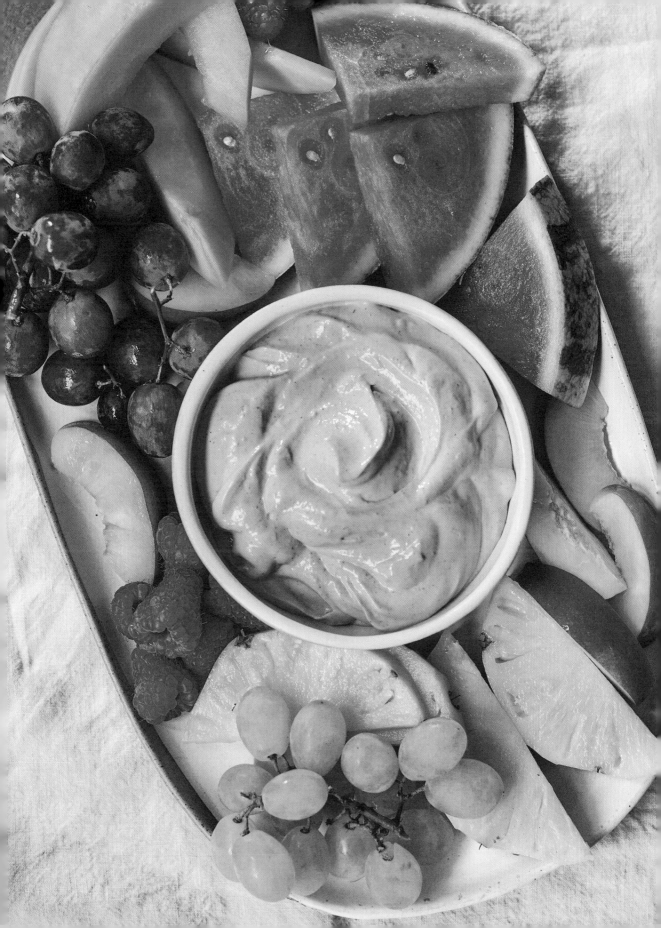

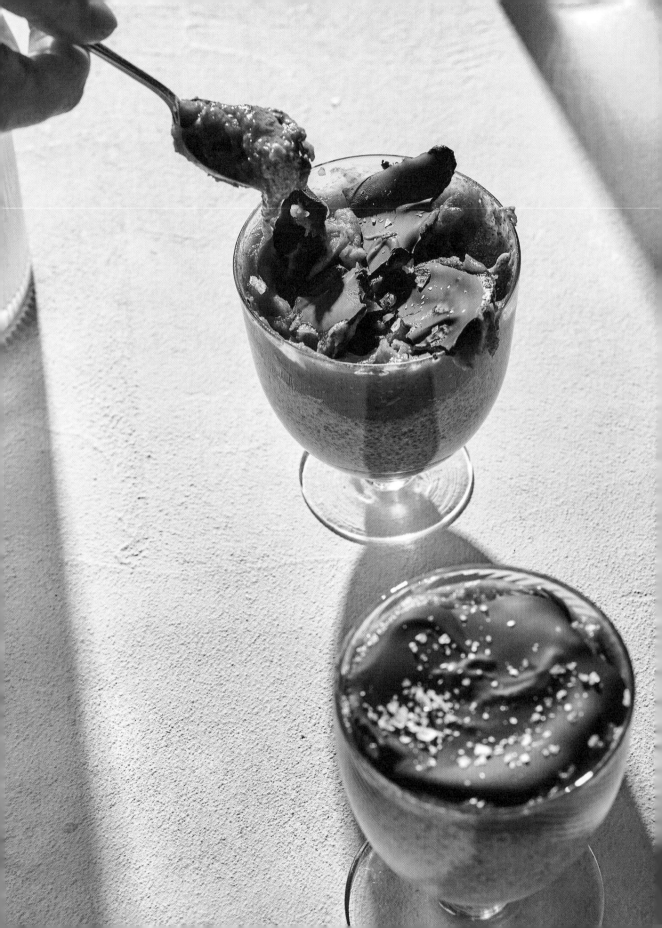

Date Caramel Chia Puddings

PP
DW
BS

You're going to want to make a BIG batch of this date caramel and put it on everything, it's so good. I love to blitz my chia here for a dessert as an alternative to the traditional chia pudding texture.

Serves 4 | Total time: 20 minutes, plus chiling

5½oz (150g) pitted Medjool dates

1 cup (250ml) oat milk or milk of your choice

3 tbsp peanut butter

1¼oz (40g) chia seeds

2 tbsp maple syrup

⅔ cup (150g) Greek yogurt (optional)

4 tbsp coconut milk

¼ tsp ground cinnamon

½ tsp vanilla extract

2½oz (75g) dark chocolate

flaky salt

Boil a kettle and pour enough boiling water over the pitted dates to cover them and set aside to soften.

In a blender, add the milk, peanut butter, chia seeds, and maple syrup. Season with a pinch of salt and pulse until smooth. Decant into 4 glasses, then top with a few dollops of Greek yogurt, if using. Smooth out the yogurt with the back of a teaspoon and put in the fridge to set.

Rinse out the blender, then drain the dates and put them into the blender with the coconut milk, cinnamon, and vanilla. Blend until smooth.

Spoon this date caramel on top of the puddings.

Add the chocolate to a heatproof bowl and melt it in the microwave in 30-second bursts, stirring regularly. Drizzle the melted chocolate over the top of the caramel. Add a pinch of flaky salt and refrigerate until you're ready to eat.

These will last in the fridge for 3 days, so they're great to make ahead.

Protein | 9.8g/portion
Carbohydrate | 44g/portion
Fiber | 8.9g/portion

Raspberry Ripple Semifreddo

BS

It may come as a surprise, but vodka lowers the freezing point of this semifreddo, which prevents it from becoming too icy, while still keeping the sugar content low. This dessert is best served a few hours after you make it—if you leave it in the freezer too long, it takes too long to defrost. Instead of using the traditional crème fraîche, I have used yogurt, since it has bone-health benefits.

Serves 8 | Total time: 30 minutes, plus freezing

9oz (250g) raspberries, plus extra to serve

1 tbsp maple syrup

1¾ cups (400g) prepared vanilla pudding

1 cup (250g) Greek yogurt

2½ tbsp vodka

Line a 9in (23cm) loaf pan with plastic wrap.

In a saucepan on low heat, cook the raspberries with the maple syrup for 15–20 minutes, until lots of the liquid has evaporated and the mixture has thickened. Remove from the heat and let cool.

In the meantime, mix together the vanilla pudding, yogurt, and vodka. Once the raspberry mixture is cool, mix a quarter of the fruit mixture into the yogurt.

Then start to dollop the yogurt mixture into the lined loaf pan and use a spoon to drag through the raspberry jam. Continue in layers until the yogurt mixture and raspberry jam have been used up.

Freeze for 1½–4 hours until softly set. Slice and enjoy with a few more raspberries on the side.

Protein | 4.5g/portion
Carbohydrate | 11g/portion
Fiber | 1.4g/portion

Grapefruit & Lemon Loaf

This loaf cake is a take on a more classic lemon drizzle cake, combining both grapefruit and lemons. The olive oil replaces the butter here, making the cake lower in saturated fats.

Serves 12 | Total time: 1 hour

⅓ cup (90ml) extra virgin olive oil

1 cup (250g) Greek yogurt

⅔ cup (150ml) maple syrup

2 eggs

zest and juice of 1 grapefruit (approx. 5 tbsp/80ml)

zest of 1 lemon

5½oz (150g) ground almonds

1¼ cups (150g) all-purpose flour

3 tbsp milled flaxseed

2 tsp baking powder

2 tsp baking soda

pinch of salt

FOR THE GLAZE

juice of ½ lemon

2 tbsp maple syrup

Preheat the oven to 300°F (150°C). Line a 9in (23cm) loaf pan with parchment paper.

In a large bowl, whisk together the olive oil, yogurt, maple syrup, and eggs along with the grapefruit zest and juice and the lemon zest.

Add the ground almonds, flour, milled flaxseed, baking powder, baking soda, and salt. Mix well to combine.

Pour the mixture into the lined loaf pan and bake for 45–50 minutes, until risen, golden, and a skewer inserted into the center comes out with a few moist crumbs.

Let cool slightly, then mix together the lemon juice and maple syrup. Brush this over the top of the loaf before slicing and serving. Any leftovers will keep in an airtight container for 2–3 days.

Protein | 5.7g/portion
Carbohydrate | 11g/portion
Fiber | 1.6g/portion

Grilled Tropical Fruit Salad

PP

DW

BS

A beautiful way to boost your fiber intake, charring pineapple and mango brings out their natural sweetness and adds a nice smoky flavor to the table. All served on a bed of cooling, lime-spiked Greek yogurt, this is guaranteed to be a crowd-pleaser.

Serves 4 | Total time: 20 minutes

½ small pineapple

1 mango

¾ cup (200g) Greek yogurt

1 tsp vanilla extract

zest of 1 lime, lime quartered

1 tbsp maple syrup

handful of pomegranate seeds

handful of mint leaves

Peel and core the pineapple and cut into thick strips. Peel the mango, remove the pit, and cut into strips of a similar size to the pineapple.

Preheat a griddle pan or large skillet and cook the fruit slices for 3–4 minutes on each side, until lightly charred. Repeat in batches until all the fruit is cooked.

In the meantime, mix the yogurt with the vanilla, lime zest, and maple syrup. Spread this on the bottom of a large platter. Top with the charred fruit and then sprinkle over the pomegranate seeds and mint leaves. Place the zested lime wedges on the platter to squeeze over the fruit.

Protein | 5.9g/portion
Carbohydrate | 26g/portion
Fiber | 2.3g/portion

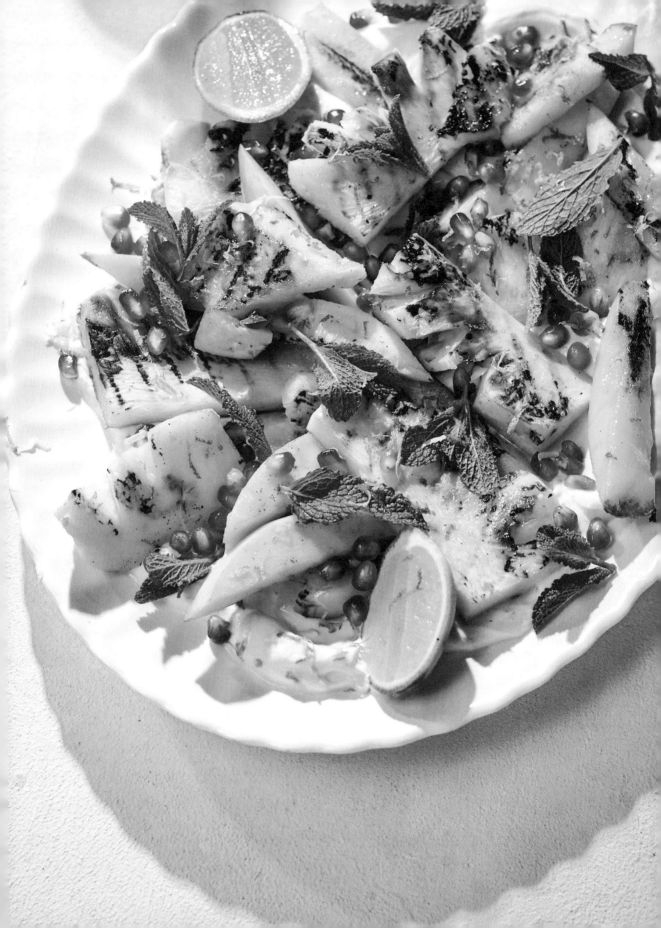

Oatmeal & Cranberry Cookies

DW
BS
WG

A little twist on the traditional oatmeal raisin cookie. The dried cranberries provide a delicious tart sweetness.

Makes 12 | Total time: 20 minutes

3 tbsp unsalted butter

1¼ cups (120g) rolled oats

¾ cup (100g) all-purpose flour

2½oz (75g) dried cranberries

2 tbsp milled flaxseeds

1oz (25g) fresh ginger, finely grated

1 tsp ground cinnamon

½ tsp baking powder

1 egg

¼ cup (65g) smooth peanut butter

3½ tbsp maple syrup

1 tsp vanilla extract

flaky sea salt

Preheat the oven to 350°F (180°C). Line a large baking sheet with parchment paper.

Melt the butter in a saucepan and set aside to cool.

Add the oats, flour, cranberries, flaxseeds, grated ginger, cinnamon, and baking powder to a large mixing bowl with a generous pinch of flaky salt.

Add the egg, peanut butter, maple syrup, and vanilla to the melted butter and stir to combine.

Pour the wet ingredients into the dry and stir to combine.

Use your hands to make 12 equal balls and place onto the lined baking sheet. Press down gently to flatten slightly.

Bake in the oven for 12 minutes, then let cool on the baking sheet. These will keep in an airtight container for up to 4 days.

Protein | 4.8g/portion
Carbohydrate | 20g/portion
Fiber | 2.5g/portion

White Bean Maple Blondies

Beans may sound like an odd ingredient, but they make the fudgiest, gooiest brownies, while being super high in fiber—a good hack!

Makes 12 | Total time: 40 minutes

¾ cup (70g) rolled oats

1¼ cups (260ml) maple syrup

2 x 14oz (425g) cans of cannellini beans, drained

½ cup (130g) almond butter

½ tsp baking soda

5½oz (150g) dark chocolate chips

Preheat the oven to 350°F (180°C). Line an 8in (20cm) baking dish with parchment paper.

Add the oats to a high-powered blender or food processor and blend to make an easy oat flour. Add the remaining ingredients, except the chocolate chips, to the blender and pulse until smooth.

Stir in most of the chocolate chips with a spoon.

Transfer to the lined baking dish and sprinkle with the remaining chocolate chips.

Bake for 20–25 minutes until the top has a smooth, crackly appearance.

Let cool slightly before slicing and enjoying. You can store these in the fridge for up to three days.

Protein | 8.6g/portion
Carbohydrate | 37g/portion
Fiber | 5.9g/portion

Cherry Pistachio Parfait

PP
DW
BS
O3

Frozen cherries are a great ingredient to have in your freezer as, once defrosted, they're so juicy and make the most amazing quick compote. You can use the granola on page 153 here, or your favorite store-bought brand.

Serves 2 | Total time: 20 minutes

10oz (300g) frozen cherries

1 tsp vanilla extract

1⅓ cups (300g) soy yogurt

1oz (30g) low-sugar granola (see page 153 for homemade)

2 tbsp mixed seeds (I used sunflower, pumpkin, linseed, and sesame)

2 tbsp finely chopped pistachios

Add the cherries, vanilla, and 3 tbsp of water to a small saucepan and simmer on low heat for 5–10 minutes, until the cherries have released their juices and have become jammy and are sticky.

Layer up the soy yogurt and frozen cherry mixture in two glasses or ramekins. Top each one with half of the granola, seeds, and pistachios.

Enjoy.

Protein | 16g/portion
Carbohydrate | 35g/portion
Fiber | 8.5g/portion

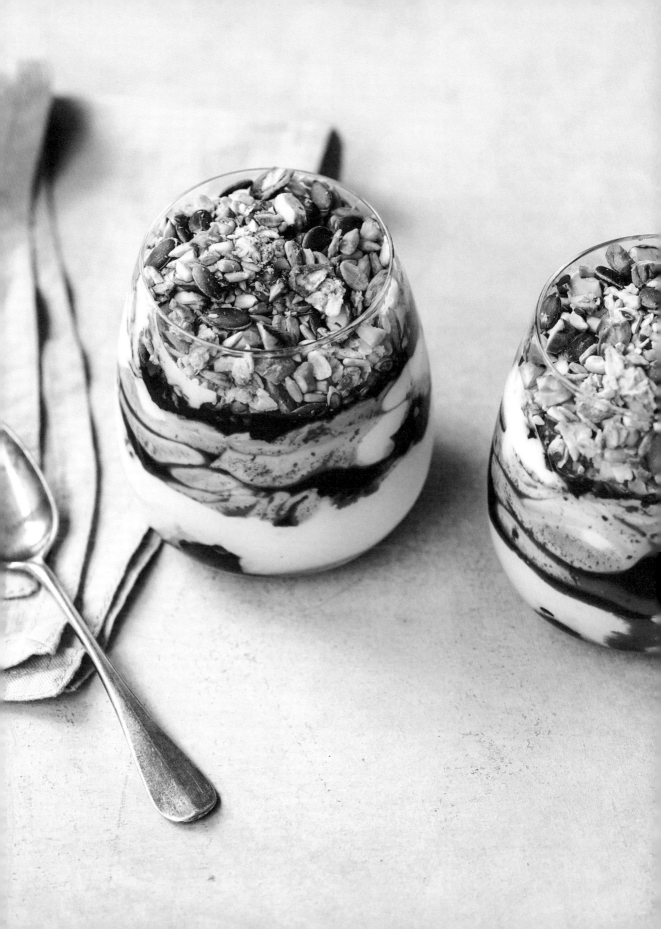

WHERE DO I GO FROM HERE?

You've absolutely smashed it! Completing my six-week exercise program is no small feat, and you should be incredibly proud of what you've accomplished.

From the first workout to the last, you've shown dedication, determination, and the ability to push through even on days when motivation was hard to find. Whether it was getting that workout done or preparing healthy meals for you and your family, I really hope you have enjoyed my workouts and realize how simple it can be to establish new habits, incorporating exercise and healthy eating into your daily life.

Over the last 25 years, I've witnessed firsthand the incredible joy that exercise can bring to people's lives, especially during midlife. This stage of life is often filled with its own unique challenges, but it's also a time when the benefits of regular exercise become even more profound. Exercise is not just about physical transformation; it's also about the sense of confidence and well-being that comes with it. In midlife, these benefits can be especially empowering, helping to boost energy levels, improve mood, and maintain strength and mobility. I've seen so many people gain a new lease on life through fitness—finding joy in movement, reconnecting with their bodies, and

realizing that age is just a number. This journey is about embracing where you are now and knowing that it's never too late to start something new, to set goals, and to achieve them.

Keep going! Remember, this is just the beginning. Fitness is a journey and now that you've laid a strong foundation for a healthier future, keep challenging yourself, whether it's by increasing your daily steps, adding more weight, or setting new goals.

As I have iterated throughout this book, the key to lasting success is balance. Keep focusing on those four fundamental pillars: exercise, nutrition, sleep, and mindset.

TAKING THE NEXT STEP

If you are ready to take the next step and be part of a community that shares your commitment to fitness, I would love you to join me on my platform: Caroline's Circuits. I have an amazing community of members from around the world, my online family who help to keep me focused, engaged, and motivated! I have four live-streamed 30-minute classes a week, all recorded so that they're available on demand, so

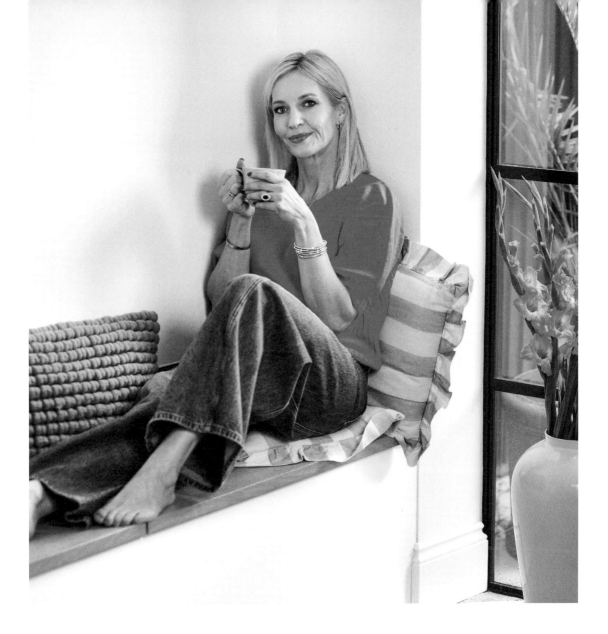

you can exercise whenever you have time. My weekly classes range from full-body classes to those dedicated to upper and lower body, core, and HIIT. I have a wide variety of classes to suit all abilities. My aim is to make life as easy as possible and ensure exercise can slot into our busy everyday schedules.

Finally, I want to add a huge thanks to you for taking this step with me in this book and laying the foundations for a stronger, healthier lifestyle. Together ,we can continue this journey and take our fitness and well-being to the next level.

Scan the QR code to learn more about Caroline's Circuits and be part of the worldwide community.

INDEX

ACKNOWLEDGMENTS

When Lauren from Bell Lomax Moreton contacted me to ask "Have you ever considered writing a book?" I was genuinely stunned. I love my job and to be able to share my passion for exercise and my experiences (specifically of strength training) with a wider audience through this first book was an incredible opportunity. I felt from day one that I was in great hands with Lauren and Callen, who both totally understood my brand, my vision and fundamentally ME!

To then work together with the incredible publishing team at DK has been such a privilege. Their professionalism and expertise have been outstanding and they have guided me through the entire process with true enthusiasm. Thank you Cara, Izzy, Jordan, and the whole DK team for making this such an exciting time. Thank you as well to Vicky and Bess for your work on editorial and design, Saskia and Lucy on recipe development and food styling, David, Lizzie, and Andrew on photography, and Charlie and Sam for my hair and makeup. A huge thank you to Laura Clark for your invaluable nutrition expertise throughout.

This book would not have been possible without my incredible family, to whom I owe a huge thank you—not only for your daily unwavering support (and patience) while I have written it, but also for your continuous encouragement and love in everything I do. You champion every single project and you always see the opportunities ahead for which I am so grateful, and I do realize how lucky I am to have you. To my wonderful children, husband, parents, brothers, and my entire family thank you for always being there. I would like to give a special thank you to my friend Harriet for your daily advice and support (alongside numerous phone calls); you have been invaluable on this journey.

I'm also indebted to my top team at Caroline's Circuits for allowing me the space to write this book while keeping the machine running perfectly in order. Lucy and Jess, thank you for everything you do, week in, week out. Thank you to my friend Flea for all of your support, too, and lending an expert eye in these final stages, which has been so helpful.

I'd like to thank the wonderful brands that I use daily and that I would recommend: The Turmeric Co., AG1, Ancient + Brave, and Symprove.

Last but most certainly not least, I need to thank my community. None of this would have been possible without the incredible members on my platforms—both on social media and on the fitness platform itself. From those PT clients I started with in 2001 to the thousands in the global community we have built today. Your energy, positivity, and support from all over the world has been incredible from the very start and we have learned so much together. It really is a positive and strong family that we have here, and this is just the start.

About the author

Caroline Idiens is a 52-year-old mom of two and personal trainer from Berkshire, England, who has taken the world of online fitness by storm—or, more specifically, by dumbbells and strength training. Caroline spent her twenties thinking that enjoying exercise meant high-intensity cardio workouts and long hours in the gym, but at 29 years old she trained as a PT, and gone were the hours of running on a treadmill, replaced instead by strength training and the positive effects it has. When lockdown hit, Caroline decided to share the benefits of women's strength training and the Caroline's Circuits community was born. Caroline's Circuits is an international online members program that focuses on 30-minute strength workouts from the comfort of your own home and is supported by 2 million followers on Instagram @carolinescircuits. Caroline and her community have been featured in *Marie Claire*, *Women's Fitness*, *Women's Health*, *The Telegraph*, *HELLO!*, *The Sun*, *Good Housekeeping*, and many more. Learn more at carolinescircuits.com

Publisher's Acknowledgements

DK would like to thank Charlie Duffy and Samantha Cooper for makeup and hair styling. Thank you to Kathy Steer for proofreading and Lisa Footitt for indexing, Martin Copeland and Aditya Katyal for picture research. DK would like to thank Saskia Sidey for recipe development and Laura Clark for the nutritional support. You can find out more about Laura's work at themenopausedietitian.co.uk, and on Instagram, @menopause.dietitian.

Picture Credits

The publisher would like to thank the following for their kind permission to reproduce their photographs:
Shutterstock.com: Omeris 2,9,10,13,14,35,43,45,49,147

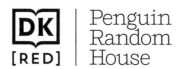

Editorial Director Cara Armstrong
Project Editor Izzy Holton
Project Art Editor Jordan Lambley
Senior Production Editor Tony Phipps
Senior Production Controller Luca Bazzoli
US Editor Margaret Parrish
US Senior Editor Shannon Beatty
Jacket and Sales Material Coordinator Emily Cannings
DTP and Design Coordinator Heather Blagden
Art Director Maxine Pedliham
Publishing Director Stephanie Jackson

Editorial Vicky Orchard
Design and Jacket Design Hello Daly
Photography David Cummings, Lizzie Mayson, Andrew Burton
Food Styling Saskia Sidey, Lucy Turnbull
Prop Styling Hannah Wilkinson

First American Edition, 2025
Published in the United States by DK RED, an imprint of DK Publishing, a division of Penguin Random House LLC
1745 Broadway, 20th Floor, New York, NY 10019

All food photography by Lizzie Mayson apart from images on pages 5, 7, 10, 12, 21, 22, 25, 37, 40, 145, and 235 by Andrew Burton
All fitness photography by David Cummings

A catalog record for this book is available from the Library of Congress.
ISBN 978-0-5939-5970-1

DK books are available at special discounts when purchased in bulk for sales promotions, premiums, fund-raising, or educational use.
For details, contact: DK Publishing Special Markets, 1745 Broadway, 20th Floor, New York, NY 10019
SpecialSales@dk.com

Printed and bound in Slovakia

www.dk.com

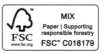